THE WAY OF HOPE

MICHIO KUSHI'S ANTI-AIDS PROGRAM

THE WAY OF HOPE

MICHIO KUSHI'S ANTI-AIDS PROGRAM

TOM MONTE

WARNER BOOKS

A Time Warner Company

Warner Books, Inc., 666 Fifth Avenue, New York, NY 10103

w A Time Warner Company

Printed in the United States of America
First Trade Printing: October 1990
10 9 8 7 6 5 4 3 2 1

Library of Congress Cataloging-in-Publication Data
Monte, Tom.
The way of hope / Tom Monte.
p. cm.
ISBN 0-446-39174-3 (pbk.)
1. AIDS (Disease)—Alternative treatment—Case studies. 2. AIDS
(Disease)—Diet therapy—Case studies. 3. Macrobiotic diet.
I. Title.
RC607.A26M68   1989
616.97'920654—dc20
89-40034
CIP

Book design: H. Roberts
Cover design: Karen Katz

for Toby,
Jacob, Christina, and Daniel

First and foremost I would like to thank the men who shared their courageous struggle with me and whose stories make up the substance of this book. I would like also to thank Michio and Aveline Kushi, whose work continues to inspire countless thousands of people around the world toward healthier and happier lives. Next, I express my deepest appreciation to Sandy Pukel, whose generous support helped make this book possible. To Dr. Martha Cottrell and Elinor Levy, Ph.D., I offer my warmest thanks for their time, guidance, and ground-breaking work.

❖　❖　❖

This book is about a group of men who used an alternative health approach as a complement to the standard medical treatment for AIDS. Nothing in this book is meant to dissuade anyone from seeking qualified medical guidance in the treatment of any illness, including AIDS.

❖　❖　❖

NOTE: The names of several of the men written about in this book have been changed in order to protect them from the discrimination routinely leveled against those who suffer from AIDS.

Elinor Levy, Ph.D.

I n 1984, when our study began, AIDS was still an altogether mysterious disease. It had first been described in 1981 when gay men on the East and West Coasts began showing up with rare diseases previously associated with a suppressed immune system. One disease was pneumocystis carinii pneumonia, an opportunistic infection, and the other was a type of skin cancer called Kaposi's sarcoma. Until then Kaposi's sarcoma, a slowly growing cancer, was reported almost exclusively in elderly men of Mediterranean background and immunosuppressed transplant patients. In its new epidemic form it was much more aggressive. Researchers soon confirmed that these subjects were immune-suppressed; most notably they had fewer than normal lymphocytes, the kind of white blood cell that is critical in protecting us from many forms of disease causing organisms. The pattern of spread of the disease suggested it had an infectious origin. Several of the earliest cases were known to have had sexual contact with one another. Recipients of blood transfusions, hemophiliacs, Haitians, and intravenous drug users were soon added to the list of those affected by AIDS.

The first breakthrough in understanding the disease came when workers led by Luc Montagnier at the Institut Pasteur isolated what they believed was the virus that causes AIDS. Their hypothesis was quickly confirmed by workers headed by Robert Gallo at the National Institutes of Health. AIDS was a new disease. Some in the scientific community were intrigued. The more idealistic saw it as a challenge and a chance to make a contribution. The more ambitious saw it as a chance to make a name for themselves. The more capitalistic looked for opportunities to make money. Perhaps the majority were disinterested or somehow suspicious of all the attention this new disease engendered, and many thought there was more hype than substance to the claims that we were at the beginning of an epidemic that threatened the health of the nation. Unfortunately, the initial response of the federal government was very limited. There was much confusion and little attempt to educate the public or those who were most at risk.

Today much has been learned about AIDS. Much of the work that has defined the complex genetic structure and functioning of the human immunodeficiency virus (HIV) has been truly exquisite, using the newest technology molecular biology has to offer. Yet much remains unknown. We still don't know how infection with this virus leads to disease, why the immune system becomes irreparably damaged, why only a fraction of people exposed to HIV become infected by it, or how to kill the virus once it has infected someone. Early promises made by the Department of Health and Human Services that a vaccine would be found within a year have not been fulfilled. Our first approaches, elegant though they were, have proved ineffective, and no one is certain that new approaches will be any more successful.

In 1984 I was given the opportunity to work with a small group of men in New York who had been diagnosed with AIDS and had chosen to follow an alternative form of therapy, a macrobiotic regimen. They felt the approach was working and wanted proof with which to convince others. As an immunologist I could provide them with a quantification of CD4 and CD8 lymphocyte numbers. These numbers were important markers of HIV progression. I could also carry out functional assays to assess how well the lymphocytes were working. At that time I was interested in doing research on the pathogenesis of AIDS. What was particularly attractive to me as a scientist was that these men did not have any secondary infections and were not taking any medications that could confound the interpretation of results. Also, although I knew little about the macrobiotic regimen, I was aware that diet could influence the immune system and the course of infectious diseases. On a personal level I was immediately struck by their courage in assuming responsibility for choosing what they felt was their best hope for survival with this life-threatening disease. I was also impressed by their conviction that their unconventional choice was the right one. They were all well informed. It was sufficiently far into the epidemic that most knew of someone with AIDS who was trying chemotherapy or one of the few experimental drugs being offered. They also realized that none of the medical treatments available at that time were cures, and many treatments had unpleasant side effects. I had my doubts about whether the macrobiotic approach would do any better but also felt no ethical conflict about helping to organize the study, as I also felt it was unlikely to be harmful. I was told it was a nutritionally adequate diet if practiced according to the advice of Michio Kushi, the foremost proponent of the macrobiotic approach on the East Coast. It was also clear that a commitment to the regimen for these men also included giving up alcohol and recreational drug use. Most also started to exercise regularly and practiced meditation and massage therapy to reduce stress. It clearly allowed the men a feeling of control over their destiny and a sense of hope. I knew all of these elements, including the low-fat, mineral-rich diet, had the potential to enhance immunity.

As the study continued, I met with the men from time to time at their self-run support group meetings to share results and answer questions about the study, new AIDS drugs, and immunology in general. Sometimes Michio and Aveline Kushi, or one of the senior macrobiotic counselors, would be there as well. I'd listen as the men went around the room, sharing both their fears and triumphs. My respect for these men is enormous. I know I learned a lot more from them than I was able to teach.

To date, the scientific community at large has shown a rather subdued interest in the study, largely because of the small sample size and the lack of control subjects with AIDS. Both these drawbacks inevitably followed from our lack of funds. Everything in New York was done on a volunteer basis. Nevertheless there has been some interest. I was very honored to be asked to testify before the Presidential Commission on the Human Immunodeficiency Virus Epidemic. I have also been able to accept invitations to speak about the study in Amsterdam, Brazzaville, Belgrade, and Zagreb. Martha Cottrell, my collaborator in the study, has additionally spoken in England, France, and Japan. In the Congo, particularly, many physicians saw this as an appealing approach because of the widespread problems of malnutrition in their country. In Yugoslavia (and I understand in other eastern European countries as well) both physicians and the public seemed very open to the idea that diet and general philosophy of life could have significant effects on health. There has also been interest from the American Medical Association's committee on health fraud. They rightfully investigate unorthodox treatments and are concerned that such treatments be truthful in their claims. Clearly there are people who are either overzealous or unscrupulous and promote alternative therapies as more effective than they are.

Meanwhile some of the participants are still doing very well. There are those who are working regularly, maintaining a busy schedule, four and five years after their diagnosis with AIDS. They show no visible signs of their illness. Others have died. Because the study was small and because people with AIDS can have diverse clinical courses, it is difficult to draw conclusions about why some men have done better than others or whether this group has done better than those who have followed more traditional protocols. Certainly they have done no worse. It has been frustrating not to have had the funding to do a larger study.

There are so many questions that might be addressed. Does the macrobiotic diet potentiate immunity in people with AIDS? How important are the psychological benefits of hope and partici- pation? Are the changes in behaviors beneficial? Do people with AIDS who faithfully follow a macrobiotic regimen survive longer than those who use AZT? Although there has been considerable clamor from AIDS activists to get the FDA to approve drugs more rapidly, none of the drugs being tested appear to offer the hope of a cure for AIDS. Perhaps we have been relying too exclusively on the medical community. Perhaps there is a lot to learn from the stories of these men.

FOREWORD

Martha C. Cottrell, M.D.

I t is now five years since I began working with these men, and others, who chose to utilize alternative healing methods in the management of their suppressed immunity and the resultant increased vulnerability to infectious diseases, cancers, and other maladies. This has been a profound journey for us all. We began our course through uncharted waters and encountered many obstacles, many dangers and fears, but we also experienced many successes and much encouragement. We learned much about this illness. We were the first to make the bold statement that it did not have to be 100 percent fatal. We were the first to offer, in the midst of despair, hope. We were the first to document positive responses from the immune system with the use of dietary correction and behavioral and attitudinal changes. These methods were cautiously referred to as "encouraging changes in the immune system among men who were on no treatment other than utilizing dietary [macrobiotic] and stress management approaches." (*Lancet*). The experiences of this brave little band of men have encouraged thousands of others to take responsibility for their condition and for their healing, both physically and spiritually. Many of them have amazed those of us who have been privileged to assist them in their struggle to live, and to live a quality life.

We continue on our journey. We continue to learn. We remain open and flexible, receptive to change, appreciative of individual needs, as we apply the universal principles of macrobiotics. Just as ships adjust their sails to shifting winds in order to stay on course, we have adjusted or changed with our ever-increasing understanding. People are doing better. Pitfalls are being avoided; the quality of life is improving. Remission is a reality. We have been a part of creating this brighter reality. These courageous men will be remembered. Those still alive will continue to chart new courses. Those who were lost along the way also will be appreciated for their contributions in raising the consciousness of us all. This experience alerts us to the toxic life-style we have created—this life-style that will not sustain life on this planet. AIDS friends have been likened to "canaries in the mineshaft." Their experiences have warned us that what we do as individuals and as a society will determine whether our planet and all upon it will survive. We must reevaluate our priorities. We must question our values. We too must chart a new course. With their example we can do so.

I want to express my gratitude to all these men for what they have taught me about life and love. I want to thank them for allowing me to travel with them on this journey. They have touched me deeply.

INTRODUCTION

This is the story of desperate men who dared to hope—AIDS patients who volunteered to participate in a therapeutic program based on an ancient philosophy and a simple diet. The program sounded unbelievably simple when compared with the complex solutions being explored by the medical establishment. Yet it was not without some scientific support. An abundance of research has demonstrated that a healthy diet and a positive attitude enhance immune function. But to the scientists who followed the progress of these men, such a program seemed to be the softest and least effective of the therapies being proposed to combat the devastating disease of AIDS. The results, therefore, were all the more remarkable. Virtually all the men who participated in the study saw an improvement in AIDS-related symptoms; several of the men are still alive more than five years after diagnosis. But for Michio Kushi, the man who guided the participants along *The Way of Hope*, such progress was not at all surprising.

In the spring of 1983, ten men with AIDS (acquired immune deficiency syndrome) volunteered to participate in a study examining the effects of a diet and life-style on the course of their disease. The program they followed was macrobiotics, which included a diet composed chiefly of whole grains, land and sea vegetables, beans, fish, and fruit.

All the men were homosexuals living in Manhattan. They were professionals, generally affluent, ranging in age from their mid-twenties to mid-forties. Before beginning macrobiotics, their life-styles could be characterized as materially oriented and hedonistic. They were concerned primarily with advancing their careers and enjoying a fast-paced social life. Each man consumed, on a regular basis, quantities of drugs, especially cocaine, marijuana, and a variety of amphetamines; each also engaged in promiscuous sex. In short, these men fit the profile of the homosexuals at risk of contracting AIDS. Like many who get AIDS, they also developed a type of skin cancer called Kaposi's sarcoma.

Several of the men had begun macrobiotics well before the study was initiated. There was little medical science could offer as treatment for their disease, especially in 1982 and 1983, and consequently they had little to lose by adopting an alternative health approach. That macrobiotics could be used in conjunction with other conventional medical modalities, such as chemotherapy or radiation for cancer, made the program all the more appealing.

The men had other reasons for adopting macrobiotics. For one thing, a growing body of scientific evidence demonstrated that nutrition played an important role in the maintenance and enhancement of the functioning of the immune system. Second, the macrobiotic diet and philosophy was an alternative to surrender. By practicing a healthful diet and a life-supporting philosophy, the men gained a degree of control over their lives, their fears, and their health. Macrobiotics gave them a tool with which to fight their disease, and it gave them hope. An abundance of scientific evidence shows the positive effects of hope and will on immune response.

The Boston University (BU) study began in May 1983. It was conducted by BU researchers Dr. Elinor Levy and Dr. John Beldekis, both of the department of microbiology and immunology at BU. Dr. Martha Cottrell, a medical doctor and director of health at the Fashion Institute of Technology of New York City, monitored the health of the men and periodically drew blood samples from each participant. The blood was sent by overnight courier to BU, where it was analyzed by Levy and Beldekis. These blood values were compared with the original tests, or baseline results, obtained at the outset of the study.

The official number of men who participated in the study went from ten to twenty. The men were followed for three years, during which time their blood values were analyzed at regular intervals.

The men were guided in their approach to macrobiotics by Michio Kushi, the leading teacher of macrobiotics, and a number of senior macrobiotics teachers from New York and the surrounding states. While the program is grounded in a sound diet, it also includes the broader principle of maintaining balance in one's life. One of the practical aspects of such a philosophy (discussed at length in the following chapters) is that it teaches one to avoid extremes in behavior that tend to have extreme consequences on health. Moderate actions have milder effects on health. The central idea of macrobiotics is that through proper eating and living, one can establish balance and harmony in all aspects of life. The macrobiotic philosophy also embraces the concept that life is everlasting and that at the time of physical death, one's life merely changes form, but one continues living through infinity.

Levy presented her findings at the Third International Conference on Acquired Immunodeficiency Syndrome (AIDS), which took place in Washington, D.C., during the first week of June 1987. There she reported that of the twenty men studied, eight had died. The rest experienced an increase in the number of lymphocytes, or white blood cells, and a diminution of AIDS-related symptoms, including night sweats, fatigue, and weight loss. Remarkably, Levy had found that the number of T4 cells had increased over time during the first two years of the study. T4 cells, which direct the immune system's attack against disease, are destroyed by the AIDS virus. In the majority of AIDS patients, the number of T4 cells steadily declines, thus rendering the immune system incapable of responding to an illness. In addition, the men had survived well beyond the twenty-two-month average life expectancy for men with AIDS. Several were alive five years after diagnosis.

This book also recounts the story of one man who was diagnosed with AIDS and Kaposi's sarcoma in July 1982. He did not take part in the BU study but followed the macrobiotic diet diligently; and at the time this book was written in the fall of 1988, more than six years after his diagnosis, he remained productive and physically active and was leading a normal life while continuing to fight his disease.

Elinor Levy's findings may point the way to the first real chance of prolonging life, or improving the quality of life, for anyone infected with the AIDS virus or now suffering from AIDS.

Moreover, Levy's work is directly relevant to every man and woman who is concerned about his or her health. AIDS continues to spread through all segments of the U.S. population. Today, approximately 66,000 Americans have AIDS and 1.5 million are infected with HIV. Those numbers will grow.

In the October 1988 issue of *Scientific American*, William L. Heyward and James W. Curran, both of the Centers for Disease Control, wrote: ". . . given the fact that the virus is transmitted through sexual contact, through the traces of blood in needles and other drug paraphernalia and from mother to newborn infant, one can envision many possible chains of infection, which leave no segment of the U.S. population completely unaffected by the threat of AIDS."

The macrobiotic diet these men followed has applications for a wide diversity of illnesses and, indeed, can be effective in preventing many diseases long before they manifest. Levy's findings suggest that there is much every one of us can do to strengthen his or her own immune system and to prevent the onset of disease. Even after one has contracted a serious illness such as AIDS, there are measures that can be taken to enhance immune function and improve and prolong the quality of life.

The current methods of treatment, including AZT (azidothymidine), do not constitute a cure for AIDS. In addition, most of the drugs currently available have severe side effects. There is no vaccine and likely will be none in this century, according to U.S. Surgeon General C. Everett Koop.

Diet therapy is neglected by most researchers today despite the abundant scientific evidence demonstrating that the immune system is dependent upon nutrition for health. Certain nutrients, such as zinc, selenium, beta-carotene, and others, strengthen immune response, making white cells more effective against disease. Conversely, the absence of certain nutrients, and an abundance of fat, weaken immune response. The studies are unequivocal on these points. However, just as scientists were reluctant to appreciate the role of diet in the onset and prevention of cancer and heart disease—even after the studies were available—many remain unconvinced of the importance of nutrition in the treatment of immune-related illnesses.

In the pages that follow, Michio Kushi offers a bold challenge to the thinking of every American. Kushi maintains that AIDS is not a disease confined to the homosexual community. The sudden advent of "new" immunodeficiency diseases—including Epstein-Barr, chronic fatigue syndrome, and others—represents yet another slide downward in human health. The human capacity to deal effectively with antagonists in the environment is weakening. The cause, says Kushi, is the daily torrent of poisons being ingested by the body. These poisons are often hidden, for example, in processed foods that are laden with fat, sugar, chemical additives, and pesticides. The diet is often deficient in many vitamins and minerals that are essential to healthy immune function.

Kushi maintains that unless rapid changes are made in eating patterns and life-style, human health will continue to degenerate and other more frightening diseases will manifest themselves among people from all walks of life.

But there is hope. The men whose stories appear in this book abused their health, became deathly ill, and still managed—through appropriate nutrition and life-style—to continue living.

The macrobiotic approach is exactly opposite to that being employed by scientists. Rather than relying on any single weapon, such as a drug or genetic clone, macrobiotics addresses the human being as an entity composed of body, mind, and spirit, all of which need to be nourished properly in order to restore health.

There is no single factor—no nutrient, no mantra, no magic—that can be gleaned from the program and placed in a pill or potion. The strength of the program lies in its totality. It is only through the transforming effects of the diet and philosophy that macrobiotics can help stimulate the patient's own healing capabilities.

The program described in these pages does not constitute a cure for AIDS. It is a multifaceted approach that can, in some people, have a positive influence on health. It may prolong life in some and improve the quality of life for others. The sciences of nutrition and psychoneuroimmunology suggest that a healthy diet and positive attitude can do much to enhance immune function, even for those who face a life-threatening illness such as AIDS.

Of great importance is that macrobiotics can be used concurrently with other therapies.

There has not been much good news in the short, dark history of AIDS. But among a small group of men in New York City, there is hope.

CHAPTER 1

Oscar Molini sat in a coffee shop on East 77th Street and First Avenue in Manhattan, keeping an impatient watch through the windows of the restaurant. He had short dark hair, large brown eyes, and a well-trimmed beard that covered a square jaw. His five-foot-seven-inch frame was trim—not the build of an athlete, but of an artist, one who cared more about his work than his food. He waited anxiously. His hands moved obsessively over a spoon and then smeared the tiny droplets that collected on his glass of iced tea. "Where is she?" he muttered. Every time someone emerged from a taxi or crossed the street toward him, Oscar's handsome face lit with expectation. But no, it was not she. He tried to get himself under control. His passionate Cuban blood, which he often referred to with such pride when he talked about his sexual conquests, was working against him now.

It was a hot afternoon in the middle of July 1982. An old air conditioner whirred from the front of the restaurant, muffling the conversations going on around him, isolating him and driving his thoughts inward to that conversation a few weeks before when a doctor at Beth Israel Hospital had told him he had AIDS.

The events leading up to that diagnosis seemed impelled by a momentum all their own. The terrible truth finally emerged after a long series of unexpected and, initially, innocent symptoms. The symptoms grew more frightening, however, and then things truly got out of control when Oscar's lover, Michael Arlington, was diagnosed as having AIDS in early May of that year.

Michael had suffered chronic weakness, fevers, and night sweats for weeks before he finally saw a physician and had some routine tests done. To his surprise, his blood samples were sent to Beth Israel for further analysis. And then the news came: AIDS. In the spring of 1982, there was no distinction being made between AIDS and AIDS Related Complex (ARC), the latter illness being a milder form of the disease. Scientists would later discover that ARC was a precondition of AIDS in which the presence of the AIDS virus existed, along with the milder symptoms of the illness. Had that distinction existed in early 1982, Michael would have been diagnosed with ARC.

In the spring of 1982, neither Michael nor Oscar fully understood the danger posed by AIDS. They had been told the disease attacked the immune system, but both believed, at least initially, that it could be treated with drugs or by building up the body with vitamins. Like many of their friends, Michael and Oscar thought AIDS was just another disease that had to be coped with by the gay community. To be sure, both of them had had plenty of experience with sexually transmitted diseases.

Oscar had had gonorrhea five times, syphilis once. This was by no means excessive among gay men in New York, and in fact he had been infected fewer times than many. That he had had syphilis only once was miraculous, in fact. Neither disease was as debilitating, however, as amoebic dysentery, which Oscar contracted four times. Like AIDS, it was spread by exchanging body fluids during sexual contact. Recovery came only after the most devastating of treatments, a drug called Flagyl, which contained a powerful poison that caused severe intestinal cramps, relentless lethargy, dizziness, and overpowering paranoia. Flagyl had to be taken for seven days to destroy the amoebas. For hours after taking the drug, Oscar suffered from irrational fears, the most persuasive of which was that he might somehow fall from one of the windows of his twentieth-floor apartment. The first morning after he took the drug, he literally crawled on the floor, holding on for dear life lest he lose control of himself and be sucked through a window and end up on the sidewalk twenty stories below. For about a month after the amoebas had been destroyed, his body and spirit were debilitated—he was weak, out of sorts, uncomfortable in some deep place that couldn't rest.

Illnesses like syphilis, gonorrhea, and amoebic dysentery were ever-present within the gay community. The risk of contracting one or another of them was like chancing the loaded chamber in a game of Russian roulette, largely because it was common to have sex with anonymous partners, and one never knew for sure whether or not one's next lover would be free of disease. Many men were simply lucky, experiencing periods of relative health and freedom from disease, while others, particularly those who were most promiscuous, were constantly ill. They depended on penicillin or some other wonder drug and between bouts of illness never gave their bodies time to heal.

Most homosexual men simply accepted such diseases as a fact of life. There wasn't much one could do, they believed, except go to a doctor and get a prescription.

Antibiotics were more than crisis intervention, however: they had become the only means of prevention that anyone thought to take. Indeed, such drugs were a standard part of the diet, and no one talked much about the negative side effects. Tetracycline was among the favorites and perhaps the most readily available. You simply got a prescription for the drug when you had a cold and then kept renewing it any time you felt the need. There was a fringe benefit to tretracycline, too: it affected the hormone responsible for pigmentation, called melanin, making it easier to get a tan. In the circles Oscar and Michael traveled, having a tan was important, especially in the winter months when it suggested that you had the means to get away for a winter vacation, preferably to Brazil, Key West, or some other fashionable place.

After his diagnosis of AIDS, Michael was asked by Beth Israel physicians to join a study group at the hospital so doctors there

could learn more about the disease. Michael agreed. He submitted to weekly blood tests and was questioned extensively
about his symptoms. His physicians encouraged him to tell
everyone with whom he had had sex to come to Beth Israel to
have a blood test for AIDS.

Michael did encourage his principal partner, Oscar, to have
a blood test, but with little urgency. Michael simply did not
perceive that he was in grave danger, nor did he view AIDS with
the alarm that it would later cause. Indeed, apart from the night
sweats and the bouts of fatigue, Michael thought he was fine.
Like thousands of others who contracted AIDS in the early 1980s,
he suffered not only from the disease, but from a dangerous
lack of information.

In 1982, AIDS was shrouded in mystery, bias, and ignorance.
The earliest cases began to surface in the United States in 1981,
when the disease was being called GRID. In 1982 the number
of AIDS cases had begun to increase significantly; by that time,
AIDS was known to be a lethal disease that was spreading pre-
dominantly among gay men throughout the United States, especially in New York and other big cities that had significant
gay populations. The word itself was an acronym for acquired
immune deficiency syndrome. It was not until 1983 that the
French isolated the human immunodeficiency virus, or HIV, as
the cause of AIDS, but scientists in the United States did not
officially recognize HIV as the cause of the illness until 1984.

By then the medical establishment had discovered that the
virus infected and destroyed the cells of the immune system,
thus rendering inert these white blood cells and other messenger cells in the immune system. The type of white blood cells
affected are called lymphocytes, subgroups of which have been
identified as having specific roles in the immune response. The
lymphocytes directly affected by HIV are called T4 cells, which
serve to direct the immune system against a pathogen or invading organism. T4 cells are like commanding generals on the
battlefield, directing other types of white cells, such as macrophage or phagocytes—huge white cells that gobble up
invaders—against a whole range of foreign objects and organ-

isms, everything from dust particles to flu virus to cancer cells. Another type of immune cells, called T8 or suppressor cells, serve to turn off the immune response; they activate when the battle has been won and the immune system should stop waging war.

HIV destroys T4 cells, which leaves the immune system undirected and ultimately ineffective against an invading organism. Meanwhile, T8 cells can proliferate. As a result, there is no immune response to disease. Thus the body becomes the perfect host for illnesses that spread unchecked. Diseases referred to as "opportunistic," such as pneumonia, toxoplasmosis, meningitis, yeast infections (called candidiasis), and other infectious illnesses manifest and spread in the absence of adequate immune response, ultimately killing the patient.

Despite the obvious dangers the disease posed, there was little if any public education concerning AIDS. The information that did exist emanated from pulpits across the country and was often couched in moralistic terms. Indeed, as Randy Shilts points out in his book, *As the Band Played On: People, Politics and the AIDS Epidemic* (St. Martin's Press, 1987), researchers were initially dissuaded even from investigating the AIDS virus because it was thought to be confined to homosexuals and therefore did not warrant the serious attention of the scientific community. Not until the French made important discoveries, including that of the HIV virus, did researchers in the United States, whose prestige was now threatened, begin to take it seriously. Meanwhile, religious leaders from coast to coast made headlines condemning those who suffered with AIDS as moral deviants and victims of the wrath of God. This had the effect of slowing any understanding of the disease and kept the heterosexual world under the delusion that it was essentially safe from AIDS.

The absence of public information changed almost overnight, beginning in 1985 when Rock Hudson died of AIDS. The nation watched in sorrow as Hudson, the beloved symbol of American manhood, wasted away, providing a torturous education and a kind of *participation mystique* in the horrors of

AIDS. Suddenly everyone knew what AIDS did to people. The media turned their full attention to what was now being called the "AIDS epidemic."

After Hudson died, a series of deaths occurred that were attributed to AIDS-infected blood being used in transfusions at hospitals. The possibility that the nation's blood supply was unsafe brought the threat of AIDS to everyone, regardless of sexual preference. Now the true nature of the disease was clear. By 1986 the word most often used to describe the public attitude toward AIDS was "hysteria." Education campaigns shifted into high gear, warning everyone from the third grade onward of the dangers of "unsafe sex" and random use of intravenous drug needles.

But in the early spring of 1982, Oscar and Michael were still blissfully under the spell of a lethal ignorance. That ignorance could not have had a more suitable foil than Michael, whose overwhelming optimism refused to let him look at the darker side of anything in life. Michael was a sensitive and fun-loving soul who bounced around as a bartender, travel agent, and florist. More than anything else, he loved to travel, especially to the Caribbean, Mexico, or South America—anyplace where the sun was strong and could provide him with a deep tan. At twenty-nine years of age, the six-foot-one-inch former high school swimmer possessed the physique of a top athlete. He never seemed to worry about anything; there were few things a good party couldn't cure. Beneath his optimistic and playful persona, however, lay a dark belief that he would not live much past forty. It was this very conviction that drove Michael to periodic reck-lessness with drugs and sex. His attitude was that even if there were consequences to such behavior, well, there wasn't much point in getting overly concerned—life was too short.

Still, he did pass on to Oscar the advice of Beth Israel physicians to come in and have a blood test. Oscar resisted Michael's suggestion, partly because he already had noticed telltale signs of trouble. A few months earlier he had found a strange sore on his shin. At first he thought it was a bruise, probably from bumping his shin against the coffee table. But as the weeks went by, there was no evidence that the bruise was healing. He had been feeling weak lately, too. He seemed to be in the grip of some general malaise that he could not specifically define, except that he was moody and tired quickly. There was more. Oscar, who was raised in Miami, Florida, had known a young man there who had contracted AIDS and died a horrible death less than a year before. He didn't know many of the details, nor did he know the man well, but mutual friends had mentioned the man and his mysterious disease to Oscar. Now, the memory of that man and the scant details of his illness often passed in and out of Oscar's mind. He tried to put off going to Beth Israel for tests, but he felt haunted by the doctor's call.

His response was to bury himself in his work. Oscar was a successful interior designer, a graduate of Pratt Institute in New York, and a former part owner of a large showroom for interiors and furniture, which he had recently sold. While only in his mid-thirties, Molini was handling the interior designs for some of the top architects in Manhattan. He was a rising star among interior artists, and his career was the central focus of his life. Many of the people he associated with and most of the social engagements he attended were related in one way or another to getting ahead in his profession. He considered it a necessary part of business to be at the right parties or among the right people. And his dedication was paying off. The interiors of some of Manhattan's largest and most expensive new buildings, as well as the showrooms for Givenchy and Celanese, were Molini-designed. In addition, he was teaching at Parsons School of Design in New York and gaining a reputation as one of the leading young designers in the city.

It was a demanding life, but Oscar loved it. He showed up at his office each morning with an unbridled excitement for the drawings that lay waiting for him on his art boards. They were his children; he conceived them on these drawing boards and labored for weeks and months to bring them to perfection.

But now that voice from his unconscious was compelling him to answer the question that had begun to nag and frighten him: Did he have AIDS?

During the first week in June, Oscar made an appointment to see Dr. Roger Enlow, a physician at Beth Israel who was part of a team of researchers studying AIDS. Enlow had an office at Beth Israel; there he examined Oscar, prescribed a series of blood tests, and took a small biopsy of the bruise on his leg. A week later Oscar returned to the office, at which time Enlow told him that he had AIDS. His lymphocyte count was 900, perilously below the normal range of 1500 to 3500.

There was more. The lesion on his leg might be malignant; that was the preliminary finding from the first biopsy. But Enlow wanted to be certain: the lesion should be removed entirely and sent to the Centers for Disease Control (CDC) in Atlanta, Georgia, where it could be accurately assayed. This second, larger biopsy would require surgery at Beth Israel. Enlow recommended a surgeon with whom Oscar would have to make immediate arrangements.

There was nothing else to do until after the second biopsy was performed, Enlow said.

Oscar immediately called the surgeon and arranged for the operation to be performed a week later at Beth Israel. The third week in June, doctors removed the lesion and sent it to the CDC.

Another week passed. Oscar spent it in a daze, hope and fear locked in a mortal struggle within him. What if I have cancer? he kept saying to himself. No, I can't have cancer—I'm only thirty-five years old!

Finally, Dr. Enlow called with the CDC diagnosis. "You have AIDS and cancer," he told Oscar.

Specifically, he had a type of cancer called Kaposi's sarcoma, which was often associated with AIDS. Enlow asked him to come to the office. There, he gave Oscar a thick sheaf of medical articles about AIDS and told him to read the material; it would help him understand his disease.

The doctor said that there was no effective treatment for AIDS or for restoring the immune system. The best thing was to treat the cancer with chemotherapy. Enlow recommended that Oscar undergo a series of tests at Beth Israel and then begin the chemotherapy protocol.

Oscar was in shock. As the physician spoke, Oscar's armpits and feet tingled with fear. An emotional explosion inside him made Enlow's matter-of-fact voice sound as if it were coming from somewhere far away.

Quietly, Enlow suggested that it would be prudent for Oscar to put his affairs in order.

Oscar went back to work. The drawings that lay on his art boards now seemed strangely lifeless, even dead. He called a friend and told him the news. Oscar noted how calmly he was able to speak about his condition. He was holding up under the strain. He was being strong, he thought.

That night he went home and told Michael of the diagnosis. As he spoke, the absolute gravity of his situation hit him. AIDS was a mystery, but he knew what cancer meant. He was dying. He faced the terrible reality of cancer. He had seen what chemotherapy did to people. They lost their hair; their gums bled; their teeth fell out; they convulsed with fever and cold; they wasted away. Chemotherapy *was* cancer.

AIDS could be reckoned with, Oscar thought, but you died from the big C.

That night a small group of friends came over to Oscar's apartment to console him. Oscar and Michael and five friends sat in the living room and discussed the possible options. Every alternative would have to be examined, they decided. Someone suggested that Oscar go to Switzerland for a full blood transfusion. After all, AIDS and cancer were illnesses of the blood; change the blood and you should be rid of the disease. That idea carried the night and gave everyone hope. But when his friends left, Oscar fell into depression and hopelessness. His enthusiasm for traveling to some miraculous clinic in Switzerland had evaporated.

The next few weeks he explored alternative cancer therapies and made tentative inquiries into the subject of AIDS. The more Oscar learned about AIDS, the more frightened he became. He began to see why his doctor was so pessimistic about his chances. The bulk of his information came from the sheaf of articles given to him by Dr. Enlow, most of which he didn't understand. Eventually he avoided the subject of AIDS and concentrated instead on the cancer.

Most of the alternative therapies, Oscar discovered, required residence at clinics in Mexico, Switzerland, or the Bahamas. Not much information was available about these places, though, and the thought of packing up and flying off to a strange country frightened him.

The proximity of death was having its impact on Oscar and his relationships. Some of his former friends refused to associate with him now; to them he was a leper, or perhaps a terrible harbinger of things to come. In any event he simply stopped hearing from some people, and once he watched an acquaintance coming down the street glimpse him and cross the street to avoid him.

A new decisiveness now possessed him. He called it his "black-and-white attitude." When anything or anyone seemed unnecessary to him, he simply eliminated that person or activity from his life. The advice of his physician to "put his affairs in order" triggered a long chain of thoughts that usually began with the insignificant, such as to whom he would leave his television set, and ended with the profound, especially the recurring question of where he had gone wrong in life.

Once again, the moralizing he had heard about being gay began to trouble him. Was this disease divine retribution for his sexual preference? Had he brought this on himself because secretly he hated who he was? Once again he plunged into the murky reaches of his psyche, swallowed up by so much doubt about the worthiness of his existence. Was he a mistake, was his life an aberration, a mole on the body of the human race? His friends and his work brought him back to the sunlight again, he bobbed up to the surface, only to plunge back down again to the depths of despair.

Meanwhile, he continued to hunt for an alternative treatment that might save him. His closest friends were looking, too.

One such friend, Mark, was a hairdresser at a popular salon in Manhattan who had a client who was very heavily involved in diet and health issues. Her name was Cheryl Hilliard, and she was something of an evangelist in the cause of healthful eating. She had told Mark that the diet she practiced could help those who suffered from cancer. It wasn't strictly a cancer diet—it was a diet everyone should follow, Cheryl had said. Mark had already begun to adopt some of the eating patterns Cheryl advocated. He ate brown rice almost daily and tried to avoid sugar and dairy products. Oscar knew little of what Mark was doing but in the past had enjoyed making fun of him and his diet.

When Cheryl came into Mark's salon in early July for a cut, Mark told her about Oscar and his diagnosis of AIDS and cancer. Cheryl knew nothing of AIDS, but she believed that virtually any illness could be helped by the diet she practiced. A few days later Cheryl gave Mark a copy of the April 1982 issue of _East West Journal_, which featured the story of a young man, John Jodziewicz, who had cured himself of testicular cancer by following a macrobiotic diet and relying on a profound faith in God.

Cheryl asked Mark to pass the magazine on to Oscar. She'd be happy to meet him and help him begin macrobiotics, she said.

A few days later Oscar was given the magazine and read the article. Jodziewicz (pronounced "Ujevitz") had a powerful story. He had undergone extensive and torturous chemotherapy and was given little chance of living beyond 1980. Eventually he decided that the chemotherapy was killing him more quickly than his cancer and decided to go to St. Joseph's Cathedral in Quebec—renowned for its miraculous cures—hoping for divine intervention. Just before he left, Jodziewicz was told by a friend about the macrobiotic diet, which might be able to help him. Jodziewicz went to St. Joseph's, an old and beautiful cathedral located on a hill in Montreal. Several hundred steps led to the cathedral above. Those who went to St. Joseph's seeking a miracle often climbed those steps on their knees. Jodziewicz followed the ritual, praying at every step along the way. During the climb, he said, he had a powerful spiritual experience in which he felt deep within him that the macrobiotic diet would help him overcome his disease. It did. By the end of 1980, medical tests revealed no sign of his cancer. Jodziewicz was well.

Oscar was moved by the article and called Cheryl to find out more about macrobiotics. Now, as he watched intently for Cheryl Hilliard through the windows of the coffee shop where they had arranged to meet, he acknowledged to himself that his desperation made him easy prey to charlatans, quacks, and true believers. Cheryl, he suspected, might fall into the last category.

She was tall, blond, and about thirty-five years old—that was all Oscar knew. But he expected the worst: an "earth mother," frizzy-haired, dressed like a peasant, and wearing—he could see them already—Earth shoes. With effort he repressed his cynicism. There *might* be something to this if the story about the young man who had cured himself of cancer was true. That slim possibility, like a little thread of hope, was, for now, his lifeline.

Finally Cheryl appeared from behind a curtain of traffic, hurrying across First Avenue and shattering Oscar's expectations with every step she took. She was tall—perhaps six feet —with long, wavy blond hair and a good figure. She was dressed in a light blazer and a fashionable blouse and slacks. She moved with self-assurance. Here she was opening the door to the coffee shop, tall, attractive, and energetic.

After they had introduced themselves, Oscar told her that he had been diagnosed just a few days before with AIDS and cancer, and that his doctors had not held out much hope. He was scheduled to undergo a long series of tests in about a week and then begin chemotherapy. He spoke with an appealing Cuban accent, smiled often despite the gravity of the subject, and gestured expressively. Oscar was a self-reliant person, and desperate as he was, he would not lose his self-respect by burdening Cheryl with his despair.

Cheryl watched him intently the whole time he talked. She liked him and even felt a kind of maternal bond with him. She wanted to help. "You're going to get well," she declared.

Oscar's reaction to Cheryl's unmitigated optimism was paradoxical. Part of him responded with, "Oh, boy, here we go.

You've really turned yourself over to the kooks." He had a strong urge to leave the coffee shop immediately.

But he liked Cheryl, and what's more, something inside him believed her.

There was no rational reason. He just wanted to believe her—that was enough, for the time being. Cheryl might turn out to be what he hoped: sincere and honest, if a bit naive and overly enthusiastic. The macrobiotic approach—which came exclusively from the *East West* article—intrigued him; he wanted to know more. He let out a long breath and said he hoped she was right.

Cheryl didn't miss a beat. She launched into a long explanation of the macrobiotic diet and way of life. She spoke quickly and enthusiastically, and Oscar couldn't absorb it all immediately. But there were bits and pieces that seemed plausible to him.

The first idea that struck him as interesting was eminently simple: The food one eats every day changes the health of one's blood. If you eat food rich in fat, cholesterol, chemical additives, and refined sugar, your blood becomes polluted with these things, Cheryl said. This polluted blood goes to every cell in the body, dumping its fat and chemicals and sugar. The cells become unhealthy and begin to degenerate. This gives rise to disease. Blood and cells that are loaded with such pollutants are the perfect hosts for disease.

The macrobiotic diet is composed of foods that are low in fat, cholesterol, refined sugar, and chemical additives. At the same time, it is rich in nutrition and fiber. This has a beneficial effect on the immune system.

Another simple idea hit home. Cheryl said that if the blood were free of pollution, cells throughout the body would begin to "discharge" the fat, cholesterol, chemicals, and sugar from the body. The cells would regenerate, she said, and return to a state of health. The healthy cellular environment can combat disease.

"Your body is strengthened when it no longer has to fight off all the pollution that you've been putting into it every day," she said. "It's all a matter of balance between the quality and quantity of foods you put into your body, and your body's capacity to deal with these foods. If you eat fat every day, it's going to build up in your cells and you're going to get sick. If you stop eating it, your body will recover. Your body can heal itself if you let it.

"You need books that explain things much better than I can," Cheryl continued. "You'll also have to go shopping for food and cooking utensils."

They left the coffee shop and went to the East West Bookstore on Fifth Avenue between 13th and 14th Streets. Cheryl led Oscar to the macrobiotic books section and began to pull books from the shelf with an unselfconscious joy, as if flashing back on moments in her own life when each book represented a unique turning point. "This was one of the books that started it all," she said as she handed Oscar *You Are All Sanpaku*, by George Ohsawa and William Dufty. George Ohsawa, Cheryl explained, had started macrobiotics after unearthing the basic principles from ancient Japanese and Chinese writings on health, nutrition, and philosophy. Ohsawa had many students, she said, a few of whom were still around. But the main one was Michio Kushi. Cheryl then handed Oscar a couple of books by Kushi: *The Book of Macrobiotics* and *Macrobiotic Way*. She continued to take books from the shelf and place them on the growing pile in Oscar's arms. Another book she treasured was *Sugar Blues*, by William Dufty. "This will tell you what sugar does," she said. Other books followed: *Cooking with Care and Purpose*, by Lima Ohsawa, George's wife; *Introducing Macrobiotic Cooking*, by Edward and Wendy Esko—"These will show you how to prepare the food." *Healing Ourselves*, by Naboru Muromoto; *Confessions of a Medical Heretic* and *MalePractice*, by Dr. William Mendelsohn—"Mendelsohn's incredible." One after another, the books landed in Oscar's laboring arms. Finally she said, "That'll get you started."

Oscar followed Cheryl to the cashier like a beast of burden, surrendering to the leader who clearly possessed his reins.

After they left the bookstore, Cheryl and Oscar agreed to

meet in two days to go shopping for food. "Be prepared to do some serious shopping," Cheryl said with a smile as she bade Oscar good-bye.

When Oscar returned home that night, Michael asked him how it went with Cheryl.

"I think I'm going to try macrobiotics," Oscar said.

"You're kidding," Michael said. "Isn't that the diet Mark follows?"

"Yea," said Oscar, a little embarrassed.

"That's the diet you like to tease him about, isn't it?" Michael asked jokingly.

"Not anymore," said Oscar. "I'm going to give it a try."

"You think it will do any good?" Michael asked.

"It can't hurt to try. I've got to eat; I might as well eat a macrobiotic diet," said Oscar. "Why don't you do it with me?"

"Maybe I will," Michael said. "As long as you do the cooking."

"It's a deal."

Two days later Oscar and Cheryl met at Integral Yoga, a natural foods store on West 14th Street. It was softly lit; large bulk barrels stood in rows, and shelves were stuffed with foreign-looking foods. The people who worked there were what he had expected: earth mothers and earth fathers, still very caught up in being hippies. Don't these people realize that this is New York in the 1980s? thought Oscar. He got a shopping cart and followed Cheryl, who had begun scooping grain from the bins into brown bags: pounds of brown rice, millet, barley, and oats. Then she turned to the beans and started loading up on lentils, aduki (also called azuki), kidney, and pinto beans.

Once again, she managed to keep up a running commentary as she instructed Oscar on each food she selected.

Whole grains are whole foods, she told him. They still have the fiber, minerals, and vitamins that nature gave them. Refined grains, such as white rice and white breads, have been stripped of these nutrients during processing. You get plenty of calories but little nutrition from refined foods.

She directed the shopping cart to the noodle aisle and placed several varieties in the cart: udon noodles, light whole-wheat pasta that was like spaghetti; soba, made of pasta buckwheat; and whole-wheat macaroni.

Then to the soy sauce. "This is tamari," said Cheryl, holding up a dispenser bottle of black soy sauce. "Actually it's soy sauce, but George Ohsawa called it tamari because he wanted to differentiate between this soy sauce and the stuff you get in a Chinese restaurant."

"That makes sense," Oscar said.

Cheryl explained that soy sauce was a fermented product, made from soy beans. Most soy sauces, however, were filled with chemical additives to speed up the fermentation process. Fermented products, she explained, have always been a staple in the traditional human diet because they provide friendly bacteria that aid in digestion of food. Chemically fermented foods, however, are not aged as traditional soy sauces are. Therefore they lack the quality of bacteria that is so essential to healthy digestion.

"This is miso," said Cheryl, moving on. "Miso is a fermented soybean paste that is used as a base for soups and sauces. It is rich in healthy bacteria and enzymes needed for digestion, also many vitamins and minerals. It's so delicious. You can make a great miso soup by using onions and wakame seaweed."

Seaweed? thought Oscar, shuddering a little.

"Seaweeds," Cheryl said as she made her way to the seaweed section, "are loaded with minerals—iron, calcium, zinc, magnesium—so many minerals I can't remember them all." As she said this, she threw several packages of seaweeds into their cart; each was emblazoned with the seaweed's name—hijiki (also called hiziki), which consisted of long black strands; arame, short black strands; wakame, leaflike; kombu, short, black stalks. "I'll show you how to cook all of this stuff," she said, smiling.

Oscar looked at the package of kombu that happened to be immediately on top of the other foods. I can't believe I'm going to eat that stuff, he said to himself.

"Now you need greens and roots," Cheryl said as she hurried along, cart and Oscar in tow. "They should be organically grown if you can get them. Nonorganic foods are loaded with pesticides and herbicides, many of which are poisonous...."

They kept on shopping. Cheryl was in her element, the grand impresario among her magical foods. Oscar was increasingly bewildered, suffering from sensory overload and the unpleasant thought of having to eat this food. They seemed to get more foreign and, to Oscar, even more bizarre as he and Cheryl went down the aisles. Umeboshi plums—a pink, pickled plum from Japan—looked downright revolting to him. He had seen tofu before and even tried it, but he was never fond of it and now wondered how he was ever going to subsist on this diet every day. But he forced himself to be positive. This food is medicine, he kept telling himself. I'll learn to like it, that's the way it is.

And so he obediently followed Cheryl and the shopping cart down the aisles and took down from the shelves the food that she said he needed. He didn't even flinch when she suggested that he buy some chopsticks, because, she said, eventually he'd prefer them over forks and knives when he got used to eating this way.

She is assuming a lot, Oscar thought.

They went back to his apartment and unpacked the bags. Cheryl then went through his cupboards and proceeded to throw out everything that she regarded as unhealthful—almost everything in the cupboards. She had warned him that he would have to get all forms of temptation out of his house if he ever expected to eat well and recover his health. But it pained Oscar to see some of his favorite foods go into the garbage. Finally Cheryl discovered Oscar's Cuban coffee. She held it up with a look of sly satisfaction, as if she were a teacher who had just caught a pupil trying to cheat on a test, and unceremoniously threw it out.

Now that the kitchen was clean, Cheryl was ready to begin cooking.

She called her husband, who arrived shortly thereafter to help her. Soon, Michael also arrived. He stood by in amusement as the meal was being prepared. Oscar watched carefully as the two chefs expertly went about their routines.

Cheryl had begun macrobiotics in Paris in 1970, when she was twenty-three years old. She had gone there as a model for the Wilhelmina Agency in New York, where it was believed that she could gain experience and return to the United States when tall models were again in demand. In Paris she developed a fondness for a little restaurant called the Wooden Bowl, which served a wide variety of whole grains, vegetables, beans, whole-grain breads, and natural desserts. She did not know the philosophy behind the food and didn't care, but one day her interest was piqued by a circular written in French that featured an upcoming talk by Michio Kushi. There was a photograph of Kushi. A few years later when she was walking down the street in Los Angeles, her attention was captured by a photograph of the same man. This time she read the material below the picture with interest. Michio Kushi, the foremost teacher of macrobiotics in the world, was going to lecture on the subject that night. Cheryl decided to attend.

She was so impressed with Kushi and his ideas that she decided to move to Boston and study macrobiotics. After she had saturated herself with the books and lectures and spent a considerable amount of time in Kushi's presence, she moved to New York, began teaching macrobiotic cooking, and met and married her husband, David, who was a massage therapist.

Oscar watched as David and Cheryl prepared the food with care. The two focused intently on what they were doing. Cheryl stopped periodically to finish a sentence and then went back to the food with renewed concentration: cutting the vegetables, cleaning the brown rice in a colander, washing the seaweed. Oscar noticed the distinct respect the two gave the food. A sense of integrity and caring pervaded everything they did.

Cheryl set out miso soup, a rich dark brown liquid with wakame seaweed in the broth and tiny slices of scallion floating on top. Pressure-cooked rice the color of bamboo, rich and hearty, was placed in a large serving bowl. A plentiful supply of steamed kale, sliced carrots, and buttercup squash, which was a deep orange, made up the rest of the meal.

A silent prayer was offered, and then the three began to eat. To Oscar's great surprise, the soup was wonderful. He said as much. "What's not to like?" Cheryl said. The rest of the meal was equally good. And then a light went on in Oscar's head: I can eat this way, he said to himself. I can prepare this food and eat this diet. So many doubts that he had experienced when shopping suddenly evaporated. The food was edible and could even be delicious!

During the meal, Cheryl asked Oscar if he would postpone the tests he had been scheduled to take. She wondered if he would also put off starting the chemotherapy—just for a couple of weeks, to see how he responded to the diet.

Oscar thought about it for a minute. Why should he have the tests or begin chemotherapy? he wondered. He had already been told that there was no cure for AIDS! The only treatment offered was chemotherapy, which promised all the comforts of a torture chamber.

"Yes," Oscar told Cheryl. He could wait a couple of weeks. Macrobiotics seemed worth a try.

CHAPTER

2

Oscar caught on to the cooking quickly. Unlike many people who have to struggle for weeks before they finally get the beans to soften, Oscar's dishes came out well the first time he put his hand to the task. He was already a good conventional cook and had no trouble preparing these new foods. His artistic nature surfaced immediately; he experimented with a variety of recipes, tried different combinations, and generally enjoyed cooking meals for Michael and himself. Soon Michael began sharing the cooking duties, and macrobiotics became a joint venture. The two shared the cooking and the books, trying to understand both the food and the underlying philosophy.

Cheryl complimented Oscar on his cooking and continued to profess her faith in his recovery.

Oscar was hopeful, too, and told himself repeatedly that he could be among the minority of patients who recover. But it was a struggle to maintain his optimism against a tide of doubt that surrounded his use of diet as a therapy for disease.

There were so many reasons to be dubious about macrobiotics. In the first place, the theory wasn't sanctioned by the medical establishment. As far as he knew, neither macrobiotics nor diet therapy had real legitimacy in the eyes of any medical authority. If diet could help people overcome serious illnesses, why didn't doctors use it? Why wasn't it recommended as an alternative, instead of being ignored? Wasn't every M.D. or Ph.D. looking for a cure for cancer, heart disease, or diabetes? How could a person like Cheryl, who had no medical or nutritional credentials, have an answer to the problem when doctors didn't?

In addition, Oscar came face to face with some real doubts about himself. He hadn't realized how conditioned his thinking was about doctors and health until he started to make health decisions for himself. Despite the fact that it was his body and his disease he was dealing with, he soon recognized that he did not believe in his inherent right to choose his own therapy. Something inside him kept asking: Who am I to say that this approach might have some merit? In choosing macrobiotics, was he again following the path of the social outcast—the outsider?

Being a homosexual had already put him outside the boundaries of what most people liked to think of as "normal." But he had gained his freedom from the judgments of straight society long ago. Oscar's sexual preferences had been clear to him for as long as he could remember. They had emerged naturally before he had known what society judged as "normal" or otherwise. Eventually he realized he was different, but by that time his sexual orientation was well established, and there didn't seem to be much choice in the matter. He resigned himself to his difference.

As he progressed through the school system of his hometown Miami, he showed no interest in girls and had no dates in the conventional sense. Soon he met other young men with the same preferences, and his secret burden was lifted. When he got to college, the only people he brought home were other young men. His parents seemed to recognize his preferences early. Oscar's father had been something of a Latin lover in his day and had fully expected his son to follow in his footsteps, but when he did not, the older Molini left the boy alone. He distanced himself from Oscar, and soon an unbreachable chasm developed between them. He never mentioned Oscar's homosexuality, even when it became obvious.

Oscar's mother, on the other hand, remained loving and close to her son. If she had a judgment on his sexual preferences, she never let on. She seemed to care more about his happiness than anything else, though she did try to get him to attend the Catholic Mass with her, which made Oscar suspicious that perhaps she was trying to save his soul. As a child, he had loved the Mass. He was drawn to the mystery of the Latin liturgy and the attitude of holiness with which the priest performed his duties. There was a profound sense of otherworldliness in the smell of incense, the brilliant hues cast by the stained-glass windows, and the holiness of the ritual. But as he got older and his sexuality became more pronounced, he became depressed and alienated by the church's antihomosexual stance and abandoned it. His mother continued to urge him to go but offered no recriminations when he didn't.

New York and its very insular gay population held out a freedom that could not be equaled anywhere else. The homosexual community of Manhattan was a world unto itself, so well supported by its own culture that many gay men never had to venture beyond it. In the 1970s homosexuals had emerged from a very private, even underground existence, to a very public and politically powerful constituency. In this environment, Oscar grew even more comfortable with himself.

After he graduated from Pratt Institute in Manhattan in 1970, Oscar took a job as an interior designer with an architectural firm. Four years later he opened his own interior design studio and a year after that a furniture and interiors showroom. His work attracted a growing number of prestigious clients. Soon he had an ever-widening reputation in New York as a successful and creative interior artist.

Oscar's progress from an uncertain youth dealing with the early rumblings of homosexuality to a successful artist comfortable with his sexual preferences was a successful journey along the path to integration. It had been a long time since he had felt like an outsider.

Now, in embracing an alternative health system, he was facing a different set of taboos; but this time his choice concerned more than sex and art, it was life and death. What had made his decision to adopt macrobiotics easier was that his chances of surviving his disease, even with the chemotherapy, ranged from remote to nil. Still, although his doctor offered only a slight possibility of recovery, Oscar felt, at least initially, a strong urge to surrender to the chemotherapy. Finally he said no. The thing that sealed his decision was simple vanity: he didn't want to die bald and withered away.

In refusing to follow the well-traveled road to the hospital, Oscar was saying he would not surrender to the pessimistic prognosis of his physician. He was now one of those desperate souls who had left the safety of the medical establishment, the great arbiter of health care. He also came to know the rejection that polite society confers on someone who contracts a terrible illness. People avoided him as if he were a bad omen. Some of his former friends kept away from him as if they believed his disease could be spread by his breath.

Others reverted to alms giving. They lavished him with things that they otherwise would never have parted with: theater tickets, gifts. People telephoned him as if it were a duty. But the veil that covers the real motive behind such giving is transparent; behind the solicitous behavior of many lay the urge to escape the fate he had suffered, and by giving to the sick these generous souls felt they were somehow protecting themselves from the evil eye of the gods.

Oscar appreciated the motive but didn't want to take part in the charade.

What he understood was the panic people felt when confronted with death. He knew the fear that propelled a person to some fly-by-night clinic in Tijuana or South America. Something held him back from such a flight. How many people were cured at such places? he asked himself.

There were others who wanted him to surrender to the hospital and die nobly, as if by going through the tortures of chemotherapy, drugs, and surgery, he might serve a kind of penance and thus be absolved from whatever sin had brought on his fate.

Was the conventional medical doctor, with all his degrees and profound self-righteousness, also spiritually superior? Most people seemed to think so.

In fact, most people seemed convinced that the sick person needed more than a mere physical cure; he needed salvation.

For the time being, Oscar was sticking to macrobiotics; for although doubt fueled his fears, he had a strange faith in it. In some poetic and simple way, macrobiotics seemed to hold a grain of truth. For reasons he couldn't fully explain, it seemed like the right thing to do.

If Oscar needed reassurance in his decision, he didn't have to wait long.

A week after he started the diet, he received a call from Cheryl. "Go out right now and buy *Life* magazine," she told him. "There's an article in it that you'll want to read."

Oscar went immediately to the nearest newsstand and bought a copy of the August 1982 issue of *Life*. Inside was an excerpt of a forthcoming book entitled *Recalled By Life: The Story of My Recovery from Cancer*, by Anthony Sattilaro, M.D., with Tom Monte, which was about to be published by Houghton Mifflin.

The *Life* article reported on Dr. Sattilaro's successful use of a macrobiotic diet to overcome cancer. Sattilaro, who was president of Methodist Hospital in Philadelphia, had been diagnosed in 1978 as having prostate cancer that had spread to his skull, sternum, spine, left sixth rib, and right shoulder. He had received conventional treatment, including surgery and estrogen therapy, after which he was given about eighteen months to three years to live. Because it offered some hope for survival, he adopted a macrobiotic diet that same year. Eighteen months later, a bone scan and other tests revealed no trace of cancer anywhere in his body. Subsequent tests, including other bone scans, continued to confirm his good health.

Sattilaro's physicians had never seen a recovery like it. Moreover, because Sattilaro was a high-ranking physician and the head of a major hospital, his story had an impact unique among medical case histories.

Oscar read the article with intense interest. The doctor had had a most conventional background; a graduate of Rutgers University and Hahnemann Medical College, he had had a long career in medicine before attending courses at Harvard to undertake the role as chief administrator of a hospital. Ironically, Sattilaro's cancer was discovered shortly after his own father had been diagnosed with lung cancer. As he watched his father wither away and finally die in August of 1978, Sattilaro prepared for his own death.

Heading home from his father's funeral, Sattilaro picked up two hitchhikers who happened to be recent graduates of a macrobiotic cooking school at the Seventh Inn Restaurant in Boston. When he told them about his condition, one of them, Sean McLain, made the unbelievable assertion that diet could cure cancer. His explanation of the macrobiotic approach to cancer sounded like simplistic nonsense to Sattilaro. But through a series of odd and seemingly providential coincidences, he began the diet and watched his health improve with every passing week. The experience was nothing short of miraculous. Finally, blood tests and bone scans revealed that Sattilaro's cancer had disappeared.

Oscar was amazed by the article. "Now, everything was aboveboard," he would say years later. "It's one thing to read an article like that in *East West Journal*, but quite another to see it in *Life*. Now, it was out in the open. For me, macrobiotics was suddenly real."

But there was another equally important aspect to the publication of that story that affected Oscar deeply—that was its uncanny timing. He needed that article, and suddenly there it was. The timing of the *Life* piece coincided perfectly with Oscar's introduction to macrobiotics. The eerie synchronicity of the events gave him a sense of being led or directed by some benevolent force; but he was not ready to delve deeply into such speculation and even turned away from it. He took the *Life* article on its own merits and put other theories aside as best he could; still, they sat there in his consciousness, like actors in the wings, waiting for their moment.

Fortunately he had his daily routine—his work and his friends—to pull him back from a crisis at the frontiers of his identity. He told himself that he would continue to eat macrobiotically and maintain the semblance of the life he had grown accustomed to. But even as he said those things, his doubts about where all of this would lead rumbled like summer lightning on the horizon.

A couple of weeks after he began the diet, Oscar decided to visit a macrobiotic restaurant in New York. There were about half a dozen such restaurants in Manhattan, all of them distinctly different. Souen, for example, which was located on Sixth Avenue, had an upbeat American flavor; Omen in Soho was a pleasant Japanese restaurant that served Japanese-macrobiotic foods; Angelica's, on St. Mark's Place, was frequented by a distinctly eighties crowd, New Wave, punkish, and upscale. There were others that had their own personalities and atmospheres. Perhaps because he was unfamiliar with any of these restaurants, Oscar chose a place in Greenwich Village called The Caldron.

The Caldron was small and made no attempt at atmosphere. One sat at a wooden table in a room bathed in mahogany light. But what gave the restaurant its distinctive character were the people who frequented the place, many of them Orthodox Jews or hippies. There was a religious ambiance so intense, it rivaled that of a temple. The Jews, with their black clothes, black hats, some wearing yarmulkes, some with curled _payess_ dangling near their ears, radiated a religious commitment that seemed almost otherworldly. They moved silently about the restaurant, made quiet, reserved conversation, and kept to themselves. Their skin was pale, their beards black, their eyes gentle yet intense. The married women dressed in muted, often unattractive cotton dresses and wore wigs or covered their hair with cloth. They busied themselves with their children while the men maintained their silent worlds or talked with other men. They were so different from the people with whom Oscar was used to dealing that their obvious commitment to religious life seemed nothing less than awesome. It was clear that religion dictated all aspects of their behavior, including their diet.

The presence of people Oscar referred to as hippies—young to middle-aged men and women dressed in the distinctive uniforms of the sixties—seemed almost complementary to the Orthodox Jews; for these people, too, radiated their own spirituality, which, if nothing else, was clearly opposed to the materialism and greed that marked the social strata in which Oscar usually moved. They seemed to broadcast their continued adherence to the idealism and social conscience of the sixties.

Oscar had seen the religious and the socially committed before, had engaged them in conversations and superficial debates, and had not been impressed with them. They were out of step with the times, he had believed, lost souls, really, unable to make it in the fast-paced world of talent and competition. It seemed to Oscar that social conscience was something one retreated to after having failed to achieve more material personal success.

But now, when he was not so certain of himself, he began to reevaluate these people. If nothing else, their way of life was the antithesis of his own.

He partied seven nights a week. On one of those nights he'd make his weekly, prearranged appointment with his drug dealer for a week's worth of mood control: uppers, downers, some mescaline or LSD, perhaps, sometimes a touch of cocaine. He liked the pretty drugs, the so-called designer drugs that gave a soft euphoria; they loosened him up without causing a total loss of control. Control was important to Oscar, but it was important to everyone in his circle. It was considered bad form to behave bizarrely or hallucinate publicly because it ruined everyone else's good time. Such behavior also shattered the illusion that drugs were sophisticated, safe, and fashionable. One episode of bad behavior was usually sufficient cause for exclusion from future parties. Oscar was always making excuses for Michael, who was often taking that extra pill and making a mess of himself. Somehow Oscar managed to keep him from being excluded from the crowd, but he didn't want anyone making excuses for *him*.

He was careful with drugs during the week because he had to go to work each morning, but his calendar was nevertheless full. He and his friends would choose one of the clubs for the night, when they had no party to attend. Studio 54, with its distinctly gay overtones, was popular on Mondays, Thursdays, and Sundays. Saturday nights were often spent at private clubs such as the Flamingo or the Saint. The Mecca and 12 West were popular places, too. One made a choice of clubs based on the quality of the sound systems, light shows, and atmospherics. The makeup of the crowd was important, too. It had to consist of pretty people on the social and professional ladder. Oscar fit right in.

During the summer, the center of the universe, of course, was Fire Island, where gay men would show off their latest fashion creations (some of them destined to appear on the racks with designer labels two years hence). Fire Island in the seventies and early eighties was to fashion what Paris in the twenties was to literature and painting.

Oscar had settled into a routine: he went home after work, changed clothes, and, if there was time, ate a quick dinner. Often there wasn't time to eat, so he simply went out immediately to a party or club. On weekends all the stops were pulled. Friday night's partying didn't start until one or two A.M. Saturday morning. He and his friends would arrive at one of the clubs, already in a state of pharmaceutically induced bliss, and begin dancing and drinking. It was important to dance for hours without stopping, but such a feat wasn't possible without more drugs.

One of the more popular drugs for dancing and sex was amyl nitrate, which was inhaled after its capsule container was broken open. The drug was originally created to help treat heart attack victims, but it soon made its way into the gay community because it seemed to cause every nerve in the body to become hungry for experience. It elevated the need for sensory gratification, making dancing and sex all the more urgent and erotic. At the same time, it made sensory satisfaction all the more difficult to attain. The gay men on the dance floor broke open the little capsules, snorted the fumes, and went off with a lover to one of the darker corners, or a bathroom, only to return for more dancing and cruising shortly thereafter. Sex was just something one did in answer to an overpowering urge, like scratching an itch that wouldn't, or couldn't, go away. As the itch became more intense and more difficult to satisfy, the partners became all the more anonymous and random. Instead of finding satisfaction, peace, and emptiness, one was tantalized by more and more desire. Promiscuity was inevitable. Some of the gay men boasted about the number of partners they had sex with in one night. For many, the daily number of sex partners ran into the double digits; the weekly count for a smaller percentage of men could reach three figures. But it was not uncommon among gay men in New York and elsewhere to have more than a thousand partners over a period of a few years. The incredible number of sex partners was made possible by the gay bars and bathhouses that were the foundation of the commercial sex industry that had developed in New York City, San Francisco, and other big cities with large homosexual populations. People there donated illnesses to one another so that they spread in geometric progression. Syphilis, gonorrhea, and amoebic dysentery were endemic in the gay community. Even if one did not frequent the bathhouses or bars, it was likely that one's partner did, or had come in contact with someone who had.

Drugs and promiscuity were co-conspirators, each one creating a greater need for the other. Many gay men in New York seemed to be driving themselves—both pharmacologically and sensorially—toward some mythical state of ecstasy. To be sure, that dream of ecstasy included a life with a loving partner, a true soul mate with whom one could have a stable and sharing relationship; but as most of the gay men searched for that perfect "other," they engaged in promiscuous and anonymous sex. Thus sex became a thing in itself, not related at all to love or spiritual attachment.

Weekends were spent in a hallucination of hunger and all-too-brief periods of ecstasy and temporary relief. Finally, time would run out. Monday was hard on the doorstep. More drugs were necessary to get oneself to work and keep going during the day. Monday night one crashed early, utterly exhausted. For many, the cruising and drug abuse continued during the week, though at a more subdued pace.

The biological and psychological effects of such a life were as far reaching as they were obvious, but those who indulged in such behavior preferred not to think of the consequences or, when they did, often laughed them off by referring to their drug habits as "better living through chemistry."

The life-style was further reinforced among many gay men by their refusal to associate with people who didn't participate. As a result, frequent visits to the bathhouses and gay clubs and flagrant use of drugs were never questioned, even by those who were otherwise highly intelligent and sensitive people.

Like his friends, Oscar refused to look too carefully or critically at the possible effects of such a life-style, nor did he want to consider any other way to live. Yet despite his efforts at repression, he knew that the fast lane was wearing him down. His work was suffering. Lately, he was having trouble getting up in the morning; he was often tired during the day, and the vitality of his ideas was ebbing. In any case, he knew that he no longer possessed the creativity that once charged through his veins. It took more effort to get out to a party, and the satisfaction just wasn't there anymore.

As he waited for his food in the darkened atmosphere of The Caldron, Oscar watched the other patrons furtively. There was no escaping the message in this place and in the last few weeks: food was sacred.

The same reverence that Cheryl and David had demonstrated when they cooked at Oscar's apartment was here at The Caldron. The people who were attracted to macrobiotics saw something spiritual or elevating in this way of life.

What had he held as sacred in his life? Oscar asked himself. "_Nada_," was his answer—nothing.

He returned home that evening and resumed reading the books he had purchased with Cheryl. They introduced him to a system of thought that was as different from his world as East was from West. The thinking and underlying values were in direct contradiction to Oscar's, but because there was an inherent integrity and unity to the philosophy, it seemed to stand up and demand his attention.

The macrobiotic view of health, as described by Kushi and Ohsawa, was the most basic and practical set of ideas Oscar would encounter in these books. But even here the philosophy saw human health as inextricably linked to the larger forces that shape nature and drive the cosmos.

According to its proponents, macrobiotics offered a diet that promoted optimal health. Made up principally of whole grains, fresh vegetables, beans, seaweeds, fermented soybean products, soups, condiments, fruit, and fish, it was essentially a replica of the traditional Chinese and Japanese regimens. But it was also influenced by the traditional foods of the American Indians (especially in its use of corn, cornmeal, and vegetables indigenous to the Americas), Jewish and Middle Eastern traditions (including such foods as chick-peas, whole-grain breads, and falafel), and Europe (including sourdough breads, certain noodles, fermented foods such as sauerkraut and pickles, and many traditional soups, stews, and other dishes).

The obvious value of the diet was that it was extremely low in fat, cholesterol, refined flour, sugar, and artificial ingredients. It also provided an abundance of vitamins, minerals, fiber, complex carbohydrates (as opposed to refined sugars), and protein. The diet didn't tax the body with the excesses typical of modern Western diets. When one compared the biological effects of the two regimens—macrobiotic versus standard American fare— one could easily see that there were many benefits to reap from macrobiotics.

The macrobiotic diet had a fat component as low as 10 percent, as compared with the American diet, which derived as much as 40 to 50 percent of its total calories from fat.

Foods rich in fat and cholesterol, such as red meat, eggs, and dairy products, begin an insidious process that eventually cuts off blood flow and oxygen to the cells throughout the body.

Fat and cholesterol cover red blood cells and make them sticky so that they adhere to one another like a roll of coins, a condition physicians call the "rouleaux effect." When the cells are thus stuck together, their oxygen-carrying capacity is reduced substantially. Also, their ability to bend and maneuver through the tiny capillaries is reduced. They become stuck in the bottlenecks of the capillaries, causing blockages and raising blood pressure. Blood never gets to many cells and tissues, thus depriving organs of nutrients and oxygen—essential elements for life. Cells die as a result, and organs function at greatly reduced efficiency.

Cholesterol deposits, called plaque, build up within the arteries to the heart and other major organs, causing them to suffocate. Eventually an artery to the heart is closed off entirely by the plaque, and a part of the heart muscle dies from lack of oxygen, an event commonly referred to as a heart attack.

If a heart attack does not occur, or if it is not fatal and the diet is not changed, fat and cholesterol continue to accumulate in the arteries, intestines, breast tissue, prostate gland, and elsewhere, cutting off oxygen and deforming cells. Carcinogens in the diet and environment act with the fat to affect the cell's DNA or genetic code. Cell aberrations can occur, resulting in prolific and unrestrained growth, also known as cancer. Fat in the intestines promote the growth of anaerobic bacteria, which produce estrogens that fuel cancer.

Sugar and refined grains provide what are called "empty calories"—that is, they provide fuel for cells but insufficient quantities of minerals and vitamins that are needed for the cells to perform their many chores. The body is forced to leach needed nutrients, especially minerals, from bones, teeth, and muscle.

Sugar, excess protein, and fat also change the pH balance of blood and tissue, making them more acidic. Sugar converts in the body to fuel, but unused fuel converts to triglycerides or fatty acids, which raise fat levels in the blood and give rise to heart disease and other serious illnesses.

Excess animal protein (from red meat, eggs, chicken, and dairy foods) gives rise to nitrogen, which further converts to ammonia in the blood and tissues. In order to deal with ammonia, a highly toxic substance that can deform cells and DNA, the body converts it to uric acid, which, though toxic, is less harmful than ammonia. As the level of uric acid increases, it crystallizes and collects in the joints, causing symptoms of arthritis and a disease called gout. The immune system mobilizes against the uric acid crystals, which are foreign bodies in the tissues. The white cells try to absorb and digest the crystals with powerful acids. However, the sharp crystals puncture the white cells, and they spill their digestive acids onto the joints and tissues, causing increased arthritis pain and greater quantities of acid in the blood and cells. As one continues to eat large quantities of animal foods, arthritis symptoms increase; so, too, do the quantities of acid in the tissues.

Triglycerides, created by sugar, also give rise to increased uric acid levels. As a result, sugar, protein, and fat increase the acid content of the blood and tissues throughout the body.

As the acid content of the blood and tissue rises, more minerals are leached from the tissues as the body strives for a more alkaline state. Kushi writes that an acidic condition is the ideal environment for viruses and bacteria to take hold and spread.

Oxygen and minerals are especially important in the healthy functioning of the immune system. As do all cells, white blood cells need oxygen to live and work. Also, the immune system needs minerals (especially iron, selenium, zinc, and sodium), and many vitamins (especially B vitamins, vitamin C, and beta-carotene) to function properly. Without sufficient quantities of oxygen, minerals, and vitamins, the immune system cannot possibly sustain an ongoing struggle against pathogens in the environment and the pollution taken in through the diet each day.

As these pollutants collect in the blood and tissues, the lymph and other immune factors are increasingly called upon to rid the body of waste. Eventually the system becomes burdened, until the immune response becomes weak and inefficient. Lymph nodes begin to swell. The lymph system is unable to eliminate the pollution as quickly as it pours into the bloodstream from the diet.

Long before a crisis is reached, the body attempts to restore health by eliminating these harmful elements. It attempts to throw off the toxins. As it does this, symptoms arise: fatigue, skin rash, swollen glands, headaches, fever, and colds.

Unfortunately most people don't listen to the body's early warnings. They view these symptoms as a recalcitrance of the body and try to attack them with drugs. Rather than change their ways of eating and living, they resort to pharmaceutical remedies that suppress the symptoms but do nothing for the underlying problem. But suppression of the symptoms is actually suppression of the body's attempt to clean the system. As a result, the accumulation continues and the immune system is weakened. The internal environment has become a breeding ground for disease. By taking a drug, one temporarily eliminates the symptoms of illness but destroys the body's only means of communicating that a problem exists.

The macrobiotic philosophy views the common cold as the body's means of eliminating accumulated waste and toxins. Mucous discharge, sneezing, diarrhea, frequent urination, and fever are efficient methods of changing the underlying environment of the blood, lymph system, and tissues. Also, the cold forces the person to rest, thus allowing the body to devote its energies entirely to the business of house cleaning and dealing with the pathogen. Though temporarily uncomfortable, the common cold serves to cleanse the system.

The consistent intake of unhealthful foods and drugs—both pharmaceuticals and so-called recreational drugs—represents an onslaught of insults to the body that eventually weaken the immune response. It becomes too weak to mobilize against a powerful disease in the environment.

Kushi and Ohsawa presented these facts in their books, but they were more than heralds of doom. They maintained that health could be recovered through proper diet and life-style. The easiest and most effective way of doing this was by adopting a macrobiotic diet.

The diet is rich in minerals and vitamins, which strengthen immune response. It is very low in fat and cholesterol, which promotes increased oxygen in the internal environment, thus invigorating cells and organs. The absence of excess fat and cholesterol causes the body to eliminate stored lipids from the arteries, cells, and organs. The macrobiotic diet is rich in fiber, which helps eliminate waste from the system and especially from the intestines. Fiber also binds with sugar, fat, and cholesterol, helping to eliminate all three from the body.

Free of toxins, and rich in nutrients necessary for health, the macrobiotic diet promotes the body's natural defenses. These books maintained that the body's defenses were eminently powerful. And even after being impaired, they could be restored if nourished properly.

His reading provided Oscar with an intellectual basis for the course he was adopting. He developed a strong belief in the essential principles of macrobiotics and began to cook his food with an almost religious conviction that the diet and his own physical resources would be enough to overcome his disease.

In the early part of August 1982, Oscar received a telephone call from Cheryl.

"Oscar, I think you should see Michio Kushi for a consultation," she said. "He can tell you better than anyone what you should be eating."

"Okay," said Oscar. "But how do I get to him?"

"I've already taken care of that. You've got an appointment with him in Boston in three days. Be at his house at noon." Cheryl gave Oscar Kushi's address and telephone number and bade him good luck.

CHAPTER 3

Macrobiotics was born of necessity—namely George Ohsawa's necessity.

Ohsawa was born in Kyoto, Japan, in 1893. The name given him at birth was Sakurazawa Nyoiti, but he took the name George Ohsawa in his twenties when he began writing. At eighteen he contracted a severe case of tuberculosis. According to Ronald E. Kotzsch, who wrote his Ph.D. dissertation for Harvard University on the macrobiotic philosopher, Ohsawa was not expected to survive. He had already lost a brother to tuberculosis, and his family expected that George would soon be dead as well.

Shortly after his diagnosis, Ohsawa came across the writings of Ishitsuka Sagen, a nineteenth-century Japanese physician who had come to be known as Dr. Miso Soup or the Brown Rice Doctor. Ishitsuka's approach to healing was based on a diet of whole-grain brown rice, vegetables, beans, sea vegetables, and salt. He had derived the diet from ancient Chinese writings, especially the 2,500-year-old work, *The Yellow Emperor's Classic of Internal Medicine*. Ohsawa followed Ishitsuka's diet diligently and within months had cured himself of the tuberculosis.

It was a life-altering experience. Soon Ohsawa was passionately studying traditional and modern medicine, philosophy, and science. Over the next forty years, he would write more than one hundred books on these subjects.

Ohsawa was much more than a dedicated student, however. He was a remarkable combination of serious scholar and reckless adventurer.

In his early twenties, he signed on with a Japanese trader and traveled the world. Eventually he settled in Paris during the 1920s and 1930s, where he wrote books and spread a message he called "macrobiotics," meaning great or all-embracing life.

Ohsawa taught that the basis of health is human nutrition. He said that daily eating habits influence not only health, but the way people think and feel, and therefore are also the basis for individual peace and happiness.

Ohsawa gained a small following of students in Paris and was able to make a living as a writer. With the advent of World War II, however, he returned to Japan and spoke openly against his country's entry into the war. Ohsawa had traveled widely in Europe and had seen what damage World War I had done to the continent and its people. He believed that no good would come of war, and that if Japan engaged in a conflict with the West, it would eventually lose.

When Japan did declare war on the United States, Ohsawa made his thoughts widely known in his writings and public lectures—actions that were deemed treasonous by the Japanese government. He was put in jail and tortured, lost as much as 80 percent of his eyesight, and fell gravely ill. When he was released from prison at the war's end, Ohsawa was near death.

He returned to his macrobiotic diet and regained his health and most of his eyesight, though he would require glasses for the rest of his life. Shortly after his release, Ohsawa set up a school in Hiyoshi, Japan, just outside Tokyo. He named the school "Maison Ignoramus" because he considered ignorance the starting point from which one could begin to adopt the philosophy of "noncredo."

Noncredo's central tenet is that one must be free of dogma to search for life's answers. It values personal experience as the surest path to truth and enlightenment.

At the same time, Ohsawa worked for the creation of a world government, a cause championed by many renowned figures of the day, including Albert Einstein, Bertrand Russell, Upton Sinclair, Thomas Mann, and Norman Cousins.

Ohsawa maintained, however, that peace depended on individual health and sound judgment, which could only be attained by proper diet and life-style. His goal was to turn his students into healthy, spiritually vibrant world citizens because he felt that personal health and happiness was the basis for global harmony. He called his world federalist group the Student World Government Association.

In early 1949 Michio Kushi was a graduate student at Tokyo University, having earned a bachelor's degree in international affairs. Early that year he received a letter announcing a meeting of the Student World Government Association at Ohsawa's school in Hiyoshi. Kushi had been writing to New York for information about the world federalist movement, but he knew nothing of Ohsawa. His only interest at the time was to find the means for achieving peace.

From his birth in 1926, Kushi lived with his family in Hiroshima, Japan, where the Kushi family owned property and conducted a variety of family businesses. When Michio was five years old, his family moved to Ishikawa Province, where his father was a college professor and his mother a local high school teacher and later a judge.

Kushi was impelled by a strong spiritual urge early in life. As a young teenager he enjoyed going to nearby shrines and sitting in prayer and meditation. In his book *One Peaceful World*, written with Alex Jack (St. Martin's Press, 1987), Kushi writes that at a local shrine "I would sit, meditate, and pray by myself for about a half-hour each day—sometimes in the morning, sometimes on the way home from school, sometimes in the evening. One day, in my sixteenth year, while meditating in the front of the shrine, I experienced a golden and silver light enveloping me. It was shining, with many radiant spirals. Surprised, I looked around and in this glowing atmosphere felt one with the whole universe. Gradually the brilliance faded. I stood up, climbed down the steps, and went outside. Then again the light returned, and I experienced all the trees, rocks, stones, and clouds around me as part of one universal spirit. At that moment I understood that everything has life and is a manifestation of God or one eternal infinite being."

Kushi returned home and later told his parents of his experience. He said he wanted to tell everyone that "everything is spirit. Everything is God."

After high school, Kushi attended Tokyo University, where he studied international law. Toward the end of the war, just before graduating, he was drafted into the Japanese army. Kushi was still an unassigned recruit when, on August 6, 1945, the United States dropped the world's first atomic bomb on Hiroshima, destroying the city and much of the surrounding suburbs.

In *One Peaceful World*, Kushi describes the events following the dropping of the bomb. On that day he and other soldiers listened in shock as a radio bulletin announced the disaster. Kushi wrote:

"In a deeply anxious voice, the [radio] announcer reported, 'Hiroshima is attacked. We don't know what kind of bomb, but terrible misery has resulted. All communication with Hiroshima has stopped.'

"Several hours later, we received another bulletin. 'If you see an enemy airplane, immediately hide. Even if only one plane, hide deeply, in shelters or behind hard, solid walls, buildings, or basements.' Before, that was not the rule. If an enemy airplane came, we had orders to go out and shoot back. But now those orders had abruptly changed. . . .

"Details of the bombing gradually became known, though the full extent of the tragedy was not fully comprehended for many days, weeks, months, and even years. The atomic bomb exploded over Hiroshima about 8:15 A.M. on August 6. At that time, the total population of Hiroshima City was about a half million, including those living in the suburbs. The blast and firestorms of the bomb instantaneously killed and injured about three hundred thousand people. Another thirty thousand people died from radiation sickness within the next few days. Today, several decades later, people in and around Hiroshima who survived the bombing are still dying of leukemia and other forms of cancer every year."

Immediately following the attack on Hiroshima, another atomic bomb was dropped on Nagasaki. It, too, brought terrible devastation. Survivors from Nagasaki were sent to Kushi's military unit for assistance. As he helped the victims off the train, Kushi witnessed firsthand the incredible human suffering wrought by the blast.

About two months later, Kushi was discharged from the army and returned home, making a stop at Hiroshima Station. He stood on the train station platform and looked out over the charred ruin that had been the city of Hiroshima.

"As far as the eye could see, burned ashes and melted steel extended from the epicenter of the explosion, miles and miles toward the north, far to the mountains, as well as toward the east and west. I could make out fields of burned ashes, twisted steel structures, and graves containing untold souls and spirits. The barren landscape was broken occasionally by a burned tree, but there were no houses or buildings standing. There was no sign of life: no people, no animals, no birds singing. Silence prevailed.

"From deep within, tears and anger welled up. Tears for the spirits and souls of the hundreds and thousands of dead who received this unexpected misery. Anger with the senseless human greed and violence which lies deeply within all of us, including myself. Sadness for the failure of humanity to realize the shining world of spirit that had been revealed to me while meditating in the shrine. I decided somewhere deep in my heart, and without knowing how I would proceed, to devote my life to realizing peace—peace for the world, peace for all people, peace for all humanity, peace for all animals, peace for all living beings. However difficult the endeavor, whatever the sacrifice it would cost, however long it would take—perhaps tens and hundreds of generations—I resolved to dedicate myself to universal understanding and the creation of One Peaceful World."

After the war, Kushi sought ways to foster peace through the creation of a world government. He wrote to leaders of the world federalist movement throughout the United States and Europe, and in 1949 received a fateful letter directing him to the Student World Government Association at Hiyoshi, and to George Ohsawa.

Kushi was impressed by Ohsawa, but partly for the wrong reasons. He thought Ohsawa looked like an "international gangster." He had a tough and worldly face, but a tender manner. For some reason, Ohsawa took to Kushi immediately. After Kushi entered the room, Ohsawa ordered all his other students out and asked his wife, Lima, to bring tea for himself and his guest. The two sat down at a table and drank their tea.

"What are you doing?" Ohsawa asked Kushi.

"I'm studying world political problems—world government and world peace," he replied.

"Have you ever considered the dialectical application of dietary principles to the problem of world peace?" asked Ohsawa.

Kushi was intrigued. He had never considered the effects of diet on the human race.

Ohsawa urged Kushi to study the effects of food on human destiny. He maintained that it was the key to world peace.

Some months after they had met, Kushi began to attend Ohsawa's study groups on a weekly basis. There he encountered Ohsawa's central thesis, the philosophy of yin and yang.

Originating in China several thousands of years ago, the philosophy of yin and yang was seen as a guiding instrument in understanding all change in life. Its application in such practical matters as diet and prevention and treatment of disease was originally recorded in what is regarded as the first book of medicine, *The Yellow Emperor's Classic of Internal Medicine*, written five hundred years before Christ.

According to the philosophy, all things in nature are differentiated by opposites: heaven and earth, day and night, man and woman, hot and cold, tall and short, north and south, east and west, positive and negative.

All opposites can be understood in terms of yin and yang, or in terms of two complementary and antagonistic forces. Yin is seen as the expansive force in nature. It causes centrifugal movement, or movement away from the center of things. It makes things loose, tall, wet, and negatively charged. In moderation, it causes things to relax. As things become more yin, they begin to separate, decay, and eventually break down.

Yang, on the other hand, is the contracting force. It causes centripetal movement, or movement toward the center of things. It makes things tight, small, dry, and positively charged.

Examples of yin things are a hot bath or an alcoholic drink, both of which have a relaxing, or yin, effect. Excessive amounts of alcohol, however, can cause an excessive yin condition whereby one's thinking (among other things) becomes loose, random, and disorderly. Concentration breaks down. A more extreme form of yin are drugs, which are said to be mind-expanding, giving rise to enormous distortions in thinking.

Salt, which causes things to coagulate, is yang. Exercises that make muscles firm and tight are yang; stress is also yang, and chronic stress can be extremely yang, causing excessive tension, tight muscles, and narrow thinking. When one is under stress, one can only think of the problems posed by life.

Extremes of either yin or yang cause sickness.

Yin and yang are continually attracting each other because each state of being is inherently incomplete without the other. Thus every extreme condition seeks its opposite to achieve equilibrium or balance.

Oriental philosophers pointed out that examples of this phenomenon are everywhere in nature. The north pole of a magnet is attracted to the south pole. Man is attracted to woman; day is inexorably attracted to night. Stress seeks relaxation.

Yin and yang bring about orderly change, because the one is constantly changing into the other; yang things become yin, and yin things become yang. For example, summer, which is yang, changes into winter, which is yin. Day, yang, turns into night, which is yin. This change does not occur until after the phenomenon has reached its peak. Summer does not turn to fall until it has reached its zenith in July and August; night does not turn toward day until the night is its darkest; the moon begins to wane when it is fullest and begins to wax after it has disappeared from the sky; the day is brightest just before the sun heads toward the horizon. All of this occurs in a universal cycle, as yin and yang exchange places of dominance.

For the Oriental, change has always been seen as orderly, even predictable.

Over many thousands of years, Oriental healers have divided foods into the categories of yin and yang. Salt, red meat, eggs, and hard cheeses, for example, are seen as yang. They cause contraction and hardening.

Fruit, milk, sugar, alcohol, and drugs are seen as progressively more yin. Fruit has a minor expansive effect in comparison with sugar, and sugar is less expansive than drugs.

Whole grains such as brown rice, millet, barley, and oats are said to be balanced within the yin-yang spectrum. Beans are slightly more yin than grains. Vegetables are slightly more yin than beans.

Fish is more yang than grain, but less yang than chicken; chicken is less yang than eggs; red meat is more yang than eggs and fish; and salt is the most yang food of all.

Because yin and yang are constantly attracting each other to make harmony, those who eat a predominance of red meat and salt will naturally be attracted to sugar, alcohol, and, in the extreme, drugs. Their internal condition will become imbalanced on the yang side of the spectrum, thus they will crave yin foods to create balance, or peace.

Stress, which is yang, will cause one to seek out yin things to bring about relaxation. The yin or balancing element can be as uplifting as a peaceful piece of music, a film, or a walk in the forest. Or it can be an attraction to more fruit, fruit juices, sugar, alcohol, and, in the extreme, drugs.

Each person is seeking balance. Meat and sugar create a kind of balance, but there are side effects. Eventually the body cannot sustain the struggle against the side effects of such a diet, and illness results.

Yin and yang can be seen interacting in all phenomena, from the furthest reaches of the galaxy to the most infinitesimal particles of matter, the atom and its subatomic particles.

Out of the yin-yang dialectic, Ohsawa created a diet that was composed of whole grains, land and sea vegetables, beans, fruit, and fish. It was essentially the diet Ohsawa had originally met in Sagen's writings.

Ohsawa introduced Kushi to the tools that would guide the rest of his life. He had made an influential contact in the United States, namely Norman Cousins, editor of the *Saturday Review*. Cousins and Ohsawa had met when Cousins visited Japan after the war. At Ohsawa's request, Cousins arranged for Kushi to go to New York and complete his graduate school training at Columbia University. Kushi would also work with local world federalist organizations in Manhattan.

In October of 1949 Michio set off for New York City, where he continued to pursue his study of international law at Columbia; meanwhile, he also researched Utopian principles in books written by everyone from Sir Thomas More to Plato.

From New York Kushi wrote to Ohsawa and his students detailing his activities with other world federalists and his continuing study of yin and yang.

One of Ohsawa's students who read Kushi's letters avidly was Tomoko Yokoyama, whom Ohsawa had renamed Aveline. Aveline had only recently arrived at Ohsawa's school and had not met Kushi, but she found his letters irresistible.

Born in 1923 in Yokota, Japan, Aveline was third of nine children born to Banjiro and Katsue Yokoyama. Her parents had named her Tomoko, which meant "God is with me."

Early in life, Aveline showed a talent for several of the fine arts, including calligraphy, painting, and poetry. She also possessed excellent athletic skills, especially in gymnastics, a sport in which she gained national recognition during her high school and college years.

She attended Teacher's College in Hamada, Japan, in 1938 and took a position as an elementary school teacher during the war years.

Like many other Japanese following the war, Aveline wanted to dedicate herself to peace but did not know how she might apply herself—until in 1950 she heard about George Ohsawa and the school he ran at Hiyoshi.

In her autobiography, *Aveline: The Life and Dream of the Woman Behind Macrobiotics Today* (Japan Publications, 1988), written with Alex Jack, Aveline says, "The purpose of the Maison Ignoramus was to become free—free of fear, free of doubt, free of anger and hatred, free of disease. The goal was to be free of everything that was preventing us from realizing our true selves and infinite happiness, and peace."

Aveline received a curt reply of acceptance from Ohsawa shortly after she wrote to apply for admission to his school, and when she arrived at Maison Ignoramus and finally met the renowned *sensei* (master), their relationship did not get off to an auspicious beginning.

"Oh, you are the newcomer, aren't you," Ohsawa said to Aveline upon meeting her at his dojo.

"Yes, I've just come from the country of Izumo," she replied.

"The letter you sent was a real waste of paper," said Ohsawa. "Next time, use only one sheet."

Aveline recalled that her letter had been "written on several sheets of elegant stationery in large, formal calligraphic hand with beautiful brushstrokes. Later I learned that he was a fanatic about paper. To a perpetually penniless writer and publisher like Ohsawa, paper and ink were like blood. They had been scarce and expensive. Over the years he had acquired the habit of writing his manuscripts on the inside of old envelopes, on the backs of grocery lists or laundry slips, and anything else that could be reused. He wrote in the smallest possible hand, often running to the edge of the sheet without leaving room for margins. . . ."

Ohsawa then turned to some students sitting nearby and asked them to assess Aveline's health by examining her face. Ohsawa had become expert in the traditional form of diagnosis called physiognomy, a means of determining a person's health and native character by the features of the face. He had been teaching the practice to his students.

"The general conclusion," Aveline wrote, "was that my face was red from eating too much persimmon"—a remarkably accurate diagnosis, wrote Aveline, who had enjoyed the sweet fruit throughout childhood. From that point onward, Ohsawa referred to Aveline as "the girl from the Izumo mountains with a face as red as a monkey's rump."

Life at Ohsawa's school could be viewed as a spiral that began with a study of one's daily diet and swirled outward to the origins and destiny of humanity. He searched the elements of human blood and the physics of the stars for clues into the two primordial forces that, for him, drove all phenomena, yin and yang.

His appreciation for the effects of food on health was limitless. Daily equilibrium in all things—from personal health to social harmony—began with appropriate diet in Ohsawa's view. He possessed an encyclopedic understanding of the effects of specific foods on individual organs, as originally outlined by the ancient sages of China and Japan. As a result, Ohsawa placed great importance on his students' daily diet and especially on the quality of the food being offered at his dojo.

"If anything unpleasant happened during the day," wrote Aveline in her autobiography, "George Ohsawa accused the kitchen. In his view, the cook was the first one responsible for the health and harmony of the entire household."

Ohsawa dressed in Western clothing and forbade his students to address him with the traditional title of *Sensei*. He instructed them to call him Papa or George. He downplayed the importance of nationality but fostered in his students an identity as world citizens. To that end, he gave each of them a Western name.

Aveline had been raised as a Christian, yet the traditions

and mythology of her Japanese heritage were a fundamental part of her spiritual outlook. The two themes ran parallel in her life, but under Ohsawa's guidance and his teaching of yin and yang, they began to merge as one.

This was one of the primary goals of Ohsawa's teachings, to understand the central truth in all the great teachings and to be able to live that truth according to one's own nature. According to Ohsawa, all the great teachers—Buddha, Lao-tzu, Moses, Jesus, and Muhammad—taught the same fundamental truth, with minor variations for their respective cultures. Their teachings sprang from a deep understanding of the Order of the Universe and the interplay of opposites. He pointed to specific writings in Buddhism, the Tao-te-ching, the Bhagavad Gita, the Sermon on the Mount, and other Christian teachings as the articulation of the Order of the Universe. For example, he maintained that among other things, the Sermon on the Mount is Jesus' effort to teach the people how one condition naturally changes into its opposite—poverty into wealth, sickness into health, yearning for truth into the fullness of understanding.

One day Ohsawa came to Aveline privately and told her that he had a new name for her. She was still being called Tomoko, or Asta, the nickname given to her by her family. But Ohsawa said that he would henceforth call her Aveline. "He said that he had made it up from 'Ave Maria,' referring to Mary the mother of Jesus, and 'line,' a common suffix as in 'Caroline' or 'Angeline.' I was deeply moved at being given a saint's name and felt I did not deserve it. But overwhelmed with his confidence in me, I changed my name ... to Aveline and have used it every day since.... After studying yin and yang with him, my own understanding of the Bible and Jesus' teachings of love and compassion greatly increased."

Nothing inspired her more than Kushi's letters to Ohsawa and his students, which revealed his idealism and commitment to his dream. Soon she wrote to him herself and expressed her desire to begin corresponding with him personally. In her autobiography, Aveline records Kushi's first reply to her.

"My dear [Aveline], we don't know when we can meet, but

I cannot forget your kind spirit. This is very strongly felt and carved like a sculpture in my heart, deeper than the Olympian gods carved the Parthenon. Our real purpose is to appreciate life in all its wonder and beauty. Let's together follow in Jesus' footsteps and observe George Ohsawa's patient, quiet, and deep teachings."

Aveline fell in love with Kushi through his letters and eventually planned to go to America to be with him. On July 20, 1951, she arrived in San Francisco and took a Greyhound bus to New York. There, she met Kushi for the first time. He escorted her to an apartment house where other Ohsawa students were staying. Soon the two were inseparable.

Once in New York, Aveline took jobs cleaning houses and worked on her English.

Kushi was still enrolled at Columbia but was having trouble with the language. To improve his command of English, he spent hours studying the Utopian principles handed down through the ages and writing long proposals for world government. He also wrote articles for world government publications, including George Ohsawa's newspaper.

Some months after arriving in New York, Aveline wrote to a friend in Japan about her observations of Kushi: "He really is someone who has deep love and wishes to save the whole of humanity. He is always talking about the fate of the world and he likes to sit American-style in a chair. Once we went to the Catskill Mountains to visit the countryside. He tried to avoid stepping on the roadside grasses and commented that we should not kill the smallest fly or mosquito. I have always loved to pick wild flowers, and he was sad when I took their lives in this way. Other times he criticizes human folly very bitterly. He is sentimental but also has this other side to him. He really wants to change the world and has confidence that it can [be] changed. I think he can do it. That's Michio."

In 1952 the two were married by a justice of the peace in Manhattan. Kushi had two rings that he had purchased out of his small budget. Neither of them fit his or Aveline's fingers. When, during the ceremony, the moment came for him to put the ring on Aveline's finger, one of the rings was wide enough for two of her fingers, the other wouldn't make it past the tiny knuckle on her ring finger. The ceremony continued without the rings; they were married, that was the important thing.

In 1955 Ohsawa, reckless as ever, ventured into the Belgian Congo to try to convince Dr. Albert Schweitzer of the efficacy of macrobiotics. Schweitzer was treating the sick at his missionary hospital in Lambaréné, work that brought him international recognition and eventually a Nobel Peace Prize. According to Kotzsch (Ohsawa's biographer), just before seeing Schweitzer, Ohsawa contracted tropical ulcers, a disease that is fatal in virtually all cases. Schweitzer urged him to go to Europe where he could get treatment, but Ohsawa refused. He saw his disease as a test of macrobiotics and a chance to prove to Schweitzer just how effective it could be against even the worst disease.

Within two weeks Ohsawa had cured himself of the ulcers and presented himself to Schweitzer, who reacted to Ohsawa as if he were mad and refused to see him again. Undaunted, Ohsawa went to Paris and continued to teach his philosophy.

While he was alive, Ohsawa was the leading macrobiotic teacher in the world. He articulated what macrobiotics was in his writings and lectures. But his writings were very much the reflection of the man: hard-edged, brilliant, and full of hyperbole. Ohsawa saw life and the universe as founded upon justice. All phenomena were the result of cause and effect, one giving rise to the other as surely as day follows night. Therefore, he saw no reason to restrain himself when it came to making pronouncements on what was possible if one followed the order of the universe. For example, Ohsawa maintained that most diseases could be cured in ten days if one ate a strict diet. His basis for such an assertion was that many of the cells in the blood are replaced every ten days; if one consumed a diet rich in nutrition and free of toxins, the new blood cells would be born of optimal health; since the blood nourishes every cell and organ, it would thus confer the same degree of health throughout the body.

But such assertions got him into trouble and nearly put an

end to macrobiotics entirely. People understandably mistook Ohsawa's writings to mean that he recommended an all–brown rice diet as the optimal way of eating. One girl adopted this diet when she was gravely ill and eventually died. Her death caused a scandal that led several scientists to call for a banning of the macrobiotic diet.

Despite the uproar among doctors and scientists, Ohsawa remained convinced of his essential message. He saw where the Western diet was heading and worked feverishly to offer foods that were as satisfying to the palate as many of the Western foods and drinks that were fast becoming popular. One of the drinks he marveled at and wanted to equal was Coca-Cola. He used an assortment of Chinese herbs, sweeteners, and other ingredients, always testing the drink and its effects on himself. However, his experimentation brought back the tropical ulcers, which he had kept in remission with the help of his strict diet. When the ulcers resurfaced, they eventually infiltrated his heart and killed him in 1966 at the age of seventy-three.

It was then that a handful of Ohsawa's students in the United States made a greater commitment to spread macrobiotics throughout the world. The two most notable teachers other than the Kushis were Herman and Cornelia Aihara, native Japanese who settled in New York but moved to northern California in the 1960s and began teaching macrobiotics. The Aiharas were instrumental in spreading macrobiotics throughout the United States, especially on the West Coast. Another was Shizuko Yamamoto, a young Japanese woman who had left Japan at Ohsawa's urgings to help Kushi in America. Shizuko settled in New York City and eventually became the leader of the New York macrobiotics community. Shizuko Yamamoto and another macrobiotics leader, Neil Stapelman, would be among the first to assist those suffering from AIDS by offering the services at the Macrobiotic Center of New York.

Michio and Aveline Kushi soon emerged as the world's preeminent macrobiotics teachers. They were the first to introduce many of the most common natural foods to Americans. Long before rice cakes could be found in supermarkets and advertised on television, the Kushis were popping brown rice on a hot iron (similar to a waffle iron) and selling their rice cakes to their early macrobiotic students.

Aveline imported traditionally made, high-quality macrobiotic foods such as miso, tamari, shoyu, and noodles and stored them in her basement. She and Michio packaged and sold the foods themselves, a little business that eventually became Erewhon Trading Company. Erewhon began as a small natural foods grocery store in Boston, multiplied into several stores, and then grew into one of the first large-scale distributors of natural foods in the United States with warehouses on both coasts and a fleet of tractor trailers bringing natural foods to stores from New York to Los Angeles.

Other natural foods companies inspired by Ohsawa sprang up as well. Before his death, George Ohsawa gave George Kennedy, a fellow student of macrobiotics, and Herman Aihara a rice-cake-making machine. Kennedy and Aihara opened a natural foods business called Chico-San, with the rice cakes as their main product. Chico-San grew into a multimillion-dollar enterprise and was eventually purchased by Heinz, Inc., which continues to produce and market Chico-San rice cakes, sold in supermarkets across the nation.

The Kushis quickly moved into publishing. They started *East West Journal*, a national magazine with a circulation of eighty thousand; wrote more than two dozen books; and founded the East West Foundation and Kushi Institutes, the latter becoming the source of macrobiotic education with teaching centers in Amsterdam, Antwerp, Florence, Lisbon, Barcelona, Switzerland, and France.

Together, the Kushis traveled the world and attracted hundreds of thousands on every continent.

Just as they enjoyed remarkable success, the Kushis endured many painful difficulties and failures. After building Erewhon into a multimillion-dollar enterprise, Michio and Aveline turned the business over to devoted employees, only to watch the company decline and eventually fall into bankruptcy. Erewhon was sold in 1983, but the Kushis had lost their first and most successful business, to say nothing of a personal fortune and a company they both loved. The decline and fall of Erewhon was the most difficult experience of their lives.

There were endless problems with their nonprofit foundation and with the relentless demands of their schedule, which sent them to teach in places as far-flung as Tokyo, Zurich, Paris, London, Boston, Miami, and Los Angeles. It was all too common for them to be teaching on three continents in one thirty-day period.

In the course of their thirty-five-year marriage, the Kushis raised five children. They were not the type to concern themselves with dates or anniversaries, however, and both soon forgot the exact day of their wedding. Years later Michio would say their marriage took place in the fall; Aveline said it was spring. Eventually Michio wrote to the Manhattan city clerk for a record of their marriage—and the exact date of the wedding—but none could be found.

Nevertheless, if a ring is the symbol of something spiritual and everlasting, then the Kushis clearly had that something. They called it a dream—a dream for a peaceful world, for harmony and balance in their lives and in the lives of others.

For Aveline, the dream unfolded in what seemed like a never-ending series of business deals, real estate purchases, and cooking classes. She opened macrobiotic restaurants, grocery stores, helped found schools, purchased a wide array of real estate in New England, and conducted more seminars than anyone has been able to count.

For Michio, it was a relentless schedule of teaching, traveling, and business activities. The dream brought them both around the world more times than either could remember, spreading the same message—now refined by their own personalities and experiences—that Ohsawa had passed on to them.

CHAPTER

4

Three days after receiving Cheryl's telephone call, Oscar and Michael were on a train bound for Boston. Once in Boston, they took another local train to Brookline, a suburb where the Kushi family lives. From there they took a cab to the Kushi house, but on the way the driver got lost. Oscar fretted, "We're going to be late, we're going to be late." The driver made several radio calls for directions. Michael stayed calm and told Oscar to stop worrying. Eventually they found their way to Michio Kushi's house, earlier than expected.

Oscar rang the doorbell, and a young woman came to the door. They entered a small foyer where the woman asked the two to take off their shoes and place them next to a dozen others already there. When they walked into the library, they were asked to have a seat at a table in a small alcove that was bathed in the afternoon sun. In a few moments, Donna Cowan, Michio's secretary, came in and handed them a set of forms to fill out and told them that Michio would be along in a few minutes. The forms consisted of a series of questions concerning their symptoms and illnesses. After he was finished, Oscar waited in anxious silence.

Suddenly, Michio entered the library through one of the

large doors and walked quickly toward them in the alcove. "Hello, hello," he said, his deep voice welcoming as he offered his hand. He was about five feet nine and wore a dark blue suit, white shirt, a navy print tie, and black socks on his shoeless feet. His large head was slightly bowed as he walked. Oscar and Michael got up, shook his hand, and introduced themselves. "Sit down, please," Michio said with a smile. When he sat down to read the forms, Oscar and Michael studied him.

Two prominent lines ran from his wide nose to his tightly held mouth. From behind steel-rimmed glasses, he glanced up at them thoughtfully with a pair of large, peaceful eyes, then returned to scanning the paper.

Both Oscar and Michael waited anxiously until Michio finished reading, rose from his chair and asked Michael to stand. He looked closely at Michael's face, eyes, and hands. He examined the sclera of both eyes, directing him to look left, right, up, and down. Then he lifted the young man's left arm and examined it carefully, paying special attention to the inside of the arm between the wrist and the elbow. He did the same with the right arm. He asked Michael to take off his socks and looked carefully at his toes and feet.

Oscar stared fixedly at Michio, whose attention was so focused that Oscar could almost feel a gravity collect around him.

Finally Michio turned to Oscar and examined him in the same way. He asked Oscar to lift the leg of his slacks so that he could examine the Kaposi's sarcoma lesion. Michio did not register the slightest alarm; he merely gave it careful attention. When at last he stood back with a faraway look in his eyes, tension gripped Oscar like a great vise around the ribs and kidneys.

"It's not so bad," Michio reassured him with a warm smile. "Don't worry. It's going to be okay."

Those words and the purity of that moment were almost too much for Oscar to bear. Tears fell freely from his eyes.

"I didn't care if it was a lie," Oscar said years later. "It was what I wanted to hear; I wanted to believe there was some hope for me."

Now Michio was all business. He told both Oscar and Michael that they could overcome their diseases if they followed to the letter the diet he prescribed. The photocopied pamphlet he showed them was entitled "Standard Macrobiotic Dietary Practice" and contained a list of foods to eat and another list to avoid. As Michio reviewed the material, he glanced up frequently to make sure Oscar and Michael were focused and concentrating. Meanwhile, Donna Cowan wrote down all of the *sensei*'s recommendations to give to them when they left. Michio went through the booklet page by page, emphasizing specific foods they should be eating.

The recommended foods were many: they included a wide variety of grains; leafy greens, such as collards, kale, mustard, and turnip greens; squash, including summer squash, butternut, buttercup, and Hokkaido pumpkin; roots, such as carrots, burdock, onions, scallions, and daikon radish (a long white Japanese radish common now in most supermarkets); shiitake mushrooms, a Japanese mushroom grown in the United States that is large, tender, and traditionally thought to contain medicinal properties; soups, especially miso- and shoyu-based soups with wakame seaweed; a large assortment of beans, including aduki, kidney, black-eyed peas, black turtle beans, lima beans, lentils, great northern, navy, pinto, soybeans, chick-peas, and split peas; tempeh and tofu, both soybean-based foods; seaweeds, including arame, agar-agar, dulse, hijiki, kombu, nori, and wakame; a small amount of white fish, such as cod, flounder, and haddock; a variety of garnishes and condiments (including shoyu); fruits, locally grown whenever possible and in season (he recommended the fruit be cooked rather than eaten raw); seeds, such as black sesame seeds, white sesame seeds, sunflower seeds, and pumpkin seeds; snacks, such as rice cakes; certain permissible spreads; and seasonings.

He suggested a series of preparations to be applied to the body, including one for Oscar's Kaposi's sarcoma lesions. He said that, as much as possible, they should wear only cotton clothing, especially cotton underwear.

Daily life-style changes must be made, he told them, his

gaze intense and serious. He urged them to create an orderly and harmonious home. They should avoid all dark, depressing, and disorderly environments, including films or events that were chaotic, emotionally upsetting, or violent. Each day they should participate in some kind of exercise; brisk walking was sufficient. They should regulate sexual behavior, avoid multiple partners, and engage in safe sex practices. Both men needed to cultivate more positive, ambitious wishes toward life and have long-range goals to which they should strive. "Be grateful to your parents, ancestors, relatives, and all friends," Michio said. "Try to help your friends. Tell them what you are doing. Help others you meet, and appreciate nature and the Order of the Universe."

When Michio finally finished, he looked at both of them and, with a radiant smiled, asked, "Okay?" He asked to see them both in a few months and told them to call immediately if they ran into any trouble. Donna then gave Oscar the notes she had made.

Everyone was beaming as Oscar and Michael put on their shoes at the door. Just before they left, Michio said, "Every day, sing a happy song. Okay? Every day, sing a song." He smiled again and said good-bye.

Oscar felt he had just had one of the most wonderful experiences of his life. Michio's last bit of advice was so poetic, he thought, a small piece of wisdom that was like dessert after a perfect meal. Not until much later did he realize how serious Michio had been about the song; but when he told others about the visit, the only song Oscar could think of had lyrics about broken hearts.

CHAPTER 5

John Angelo realized that there was something seriously wrong with him in May 1982. The strange sores on his left leg were not going away. Neither were the swollen lymph nodes in his neck, armpits, and groin. Most frightening of all, the right side of his torso, especially his right arm, had grown steadily weaker over the past few months and was now worse than ever. The muscles in his arm had withered so badly that there was little strength left in his hand. When he awoke each morning, his arm felt as if someone had applied a tourniquet during the night—the limb was cold, numb, and strangely swollen, and he had to bend it back and forth until it had sufficient circulation to function. He knew he couldn't avoid the truth any longer.

Terrified, he went to a physician who, after examining him, sent him to Sloan Kettering Cancer Institute in Manhattan. There, doctors took a biopsy of one of three lesions on his leg and informed him that he had Kaposi's sarcoma. It was not clear at the time whether or not he had AIDS, or what his physicians were calling the "gay cancer."

His was an odd case, his doctors said. The majority of men who contract Kaposi's sarcoma are Mediterranean, sixty years of age and older. John was of Italian descent, but he was only forty-seven years old. When Kaposi's manifests in men younger than sixty, it is usually a sign of AIDS. John's physician wanted to run a battery of tests; colonoscopies and bronchoscopies were among several they suggested. The doctors at Sloan Kettering were circumspect about the possible therapies available. John pressed a physician who was an assistant to the doctor supervising his case. The assistant said that interferon, an experimental cancer therapy, was what his doctor was likely to recommend, but they would have to wait for the test results to say with certainty. John went home after seeing his doctor and decided he would wait before having the tests done.

AIDS was fast becoming a terrifying specter in the lives of every gay man John knew. People attempted to speak glibly about the new disease, as if by treating the subject lightly it might not lead to the consequences that afflicted others. John was aware that as a gay man he too was at high risk of contracting the disease, but like many of his friends, he had not changed his way of living until the disease was already upon him. Now, deep inside, he knew he had AIDS, but he didn't know what to do.

He started to visit psychics for advice. Every one of them said that he would overcome his disease. Several suggested that he begin to cleanse his system and take vitamins.

The idea of cleansing his system hit home with John. For years he had been repressing the thought that he was harming his body with drugs and promiscuous sex. He had been dependent upon drugs for the past two decades: he took a lot of uppers, especially diet pills; he often took Quaaludes to counteract the uppers; and he smoked marijuana. On occasion he had used stronger drugs like LSD, mescaline, and cocaine, but his drug of choice was marijuana, which he smoked daily. He also inhaled regular doses of amyl nitrate, especially while dancing or having sex.

Taking drugs was a fundamental part of John's life, especially his social life. He felt that if he stopped taking drugs, he would lose many of his friends. To most homosexual men, especially those in the circles John traveled in, drugs were seen as one of the freedoms gays had won during the homosexual revolution of the 1970s. A new set of attitudes had emerged among gay men and women, the most important of which was that they were free to decide what was morally right or wrong when it came to the way they treated their bodies. They had been liberated from the morality of the straight world, which, for the most part, hated them. Gay men and women were determined not to be bound by guilt or repression. That was the goal, at least—freedom and peace within the context of being gay. Drugs were a means of achieving a desired mood and an escape from many darker emotional states, especially self-hatred, which haunted many gay men and women. Drugs were viewed as both a symbol of liberation and a chemical means of achieving pleasure—albeit a short-lived pleasure and one that had side effects. Still, it was pleasure and freedom nonetheless, and the attitude was "Get what you can."

Through the sixties, seventies, and early eighties, John smoked marijuana like others drank coffee; it was just something he did when he got up in the morning and, whenever possible, continued doing during the day. His sex life was full of the same excesses: strangers, most of them, discovered at bathhouses, bars, dance places, and parties. Still, all the while he was engaged in such a life, something was nagging at him from the far reaches of his mind, telling him that it wasn't working—he wasn't getting any happier—and there would be consequences.

After being diagnosed with Kaposi's sarcoma and then being told by the psychics to cleanse his body of the poisons he was taking in, John began to unlock a door in his mind where he kept many unpleasant thoughts trapped. More than a year before he had read that doctors had discovered that amyl nitrate depressed the immune system when used regularly. He had also read that the introduction of semen into the body from multiple partners was harmful to the immune system. These were unpleasant thoughts, which for a long time he had managed to ignore. Whenever he read an article that reminded him of the dangers he was flirting with, he told himself that eventually he would change his way of life—but not now, not today.

On the morning of June 21, 1982—John's forty-eighth birthday—he stood over his toilet urinating, a marijuana cigarette hanging from his lips. He was off work and thinking about what he was going to do for himself as a birthday present. He stared blankly through the small window of his bathroom and looked out over lower Manhattan. His apartment was in the twenties near Fifth Avenue, and from his window he could see the tops of other apartment buildings and the many wooden water tanks that exist as faint reminders of simpler times. A light summer breeze blew in, touching his skin. For some reason, his gaze turned downward, causing the joint to fall from his mouth and into the toilet. For a moment he felt a small pang of disappointment at the loss. Suddenly, as if possessed by some other power, he went into his medicine cabinet and took out the rest of his marijuana and threw it into the toilet, too. And then he flushed the toilet and watched the last of his pot and his drug habit spiral down into the New York City sewer system.

That afternoon John felt a strange solace come over him. He went to a Catholic church in Greenwich Village and said a rosary. He prayed for health and for a better life. He had been miserable for a long time.

For years John had been dreaming of finding someone he could truly love. He also wanted to achieve some stability and a sense of fulfillment in his life. But he could never get the two together, largely because the things he thought would provide fulfillment were really short-lived pleasures—drugs, fashions, and one-night stands. As he'd once said, he had an overpowering need to "find out the newest place to go dancing, see the latest movie, go to the newest restaurant, buy the latest piece of clothing—and in the same way, you always wanted new relationships, so promiscuity was a part of all of that."

He had hoped that he could live such a life with impunity, an illusion made possible by the easy availability of antibiotics.

"We [John and his friends] believed that no matter what illness we got there would always be antibiotics to straighten us out."

Drugs and sex without a price! he had thought. But there

was a price. Like most others in the New York gay community, John was prey to the usual sexually transmitted diseases. And like others, he simply accepted these illnesses as part of the consequences of homosexuality and took great quantities of antibiotics.

Through all the sickness and heartache, he kept coming back to Mass and hoping for solace, forgiveness, and peace. His was a love-hate relationship with the Church, because the Vatican had made its position clear: homosexuality was an abomination. But John believed in miracles and forgiveness, so he kept coming back. Now, as he said his rosary, he hoped that the Lord was more understanding than the Church and that He would somehow help him find his way out of the terrible maze of sickness and despair that dominated his life.

He left the church that day feeling better, and that night he slept on his rosary with a small glow of peace inside him.

Through the summer of 1982, John worked at his painting. He was now achieving recognition as an artist, and galleries were requesting more of his canvasses. He must continue, no matter how difficult it was! He dreaded the tests his doctor had urged him to take and searched for alternative ways of treating his disease. He prayed a lot and again saw several psychics, who told him consistently that he would completely recover. One told him that he had a lot of friends "on the other side" who were helping him. He should keep searching. Meanwhile, he tried a variety of diets. He eliminated meat entirely and ate fish, vegetables, dairy foods (particularly cheese and butter), and sugar. There were no signs of physical improvement, but as summer turned into fall, John felt a growing faith that his life was leading him toward an answer.

That was a difficult fall for Oscar Molini, too. After his consultation with Michio Kushi, he started to go through a withdrawal period that he thought would either kill him or drive him crazy.

"I went through every head trip imaginable," Oscar once said about those months. Fortunately Cheryl was there to support him through the many deep and unsettling changes. He had received a call from her shortly after his return from Boston. "Don't be surprised if you have headaches for a few days. You're giving up a lot of coffee and drugs, you know," she told him. "Your body has to adjust to that." As she forecast, Oscar suffered for weeks with raging headaches that he thought would blow off the top of his head.

Cheryl talked a lot about "discharging," explaining the macrobiotic view that if one consumed a clean and healthy diet, the body would throw off toxins that had been accumulating over many years. "You may develop a rash or get some kind of strange skin discharge," Cheryl warned. Sure enough, within weeks Oscar developed a skin rash and a strange set of eruptions on various parts of his body, including his face, legs, and hands. He had several wicked colds and fevers, too.

There were emotional eruptions as well. For reasons he couldn't explain later, he would react intensely in situations that in the past he would have been able to handle with outward calm. He was by nature a placid person, but as fall turned into winter, he was "discharging" like a crazy man.

Some of the physical discharges clearly frightened him. He was afraid that the cancer was getting worse and that the skin eruptions were merely new forms of the Kaposi's sarcoma lesions that were already in evidence before he'd begun macrobiotics. Several times he wanted to call Michio. But for what? he asked himself. A pimple? Instead he called Cheryl, who always managed to calm him down and sometimes even congratulated him on the purity of his diet, telling him he was having such powerful reactions because his eating habits were so good. His body was eliminating a lot of accumulated poisons as quickly and efficiently as it knew how. Trust your body, she told him. The discharges would pass.

Eventually, the intensity of the discharges did indeed modulate. Oscar stopped having colds and bizarre skin eruptions. He even gained an emotional equilibrium.

More remarkable was the fact that his blood tests were

showing a dramatic improvement in his immune system. Lymphocytes, which are so essential a part of the immune system, are like soldiers, bounding down on and routing the foreign invader. When infected with the AIDS virus, however, they fail to activate in the presence of a pathogen. Once the AIDS virus has invaded the system, therefore, the number of lymphocytes in the bloodstream steadily diminishes, and those that remain are ineffective against the disease. Eventually one no longer has a sufficient number of lymphocytes to fight off one of a variety of "opportunistic" diseases. At that point an illness such as pneumonia can easily take hold in the lungs and spread until it destroys the patient.

Rather than becoming fewer in number, Oscar's lymphocyte count was rising. His physician was amazed.

"I kept telling him that I was practicing this diet and feeling better, but he did not believe me," said Oscar. "He couldn't explain why my lymphocyte count was rising."

Oscar now had great reserves of energy. He slept soundly at night. He awoke in the morning fully awake, and he was full of vitality throughout the day. At night he felt tired and had no trouble getting to sleep.

Despite the terrors of his disease, Oscar felt a growing confidence and, indeed, a deep sense of well-being. He now turned to his job with a renewed vitality and creativity. A strong wind was once again in his sails.

Meanwhile, John Angelo was getting closer to death. In the spring of 1983 he was consumed by his illness. The right side of his body had continued to deteriorate. He was so weak that he could not produce his art any longer. As a result his income was drying up. John had Blue Cross-Blue Shield benefits but did not apply for them because he was afraid that if he went through with the tests, he was certain to be diagnosed with AIDS, which would remain on his medical record and ruin any future he had left.

By the spring of 1983, AIDS was regarded by many as the next Black Plague, but because it had initially taken hold within the gay community, ministers, social commentators, and even political leaders were viewing the epidemic as a scourge set loose upon innocent people by homosexuals. Some political leaders, most notably Jesse Helms (D-N.C.), and clergy members would eventually call for a quarantine of AIDS patients in order to protect the rest of American society from the disease.

John could see it all coming and feared being segregated from society, led to a kind of leper colony and left to die. He managed to get some disability benefits without jeopardizing himself, but they were too little to cover his sizable rent and living expenses. As a result, he was now near bankruptcy.

Other issues were pressing him as well. He had begun to question his approach to finding an answer to his illness, or more accurately, his lack of an approach. His search for an appropriate therapy had degenerated into an irrational hope that by wandering along he would somehow bump into the right treatment. Meanwhile, certain questions kept nagging him. Why was he waiting? he asked himself. Waiting only allowed the illness to progress, perhaps making it impossible to stop even if he found the right answer. Wasn't nipping the disease in the bud the right thing to do? Hadn't he heard that enough already? But there was no cure for Kaposi's sarcoma, much less AIDS. John had read about interferon, which many researchers viewed with suspicion and no one regarded as a cure. He was afraid to turn to his doctors and afraid of committing himself to the alternatives he had heard about because none of them had struck him as correct. But he was flirting with death now, and he knew it. Waiting was tantamount to giving the disease a free hand.

And then fate brought John around the corner.

In May of 1983, he gave a birthday party for a friend at a Manhattan restaurant. One of the guests was a woman he had known for years, a radio and television reporter. The little gathering sat at a long table, John and the reporter sitting opposite each other. Everyone made light conversation, and jokes were flying back and forth. Food was brought, and the conversations separated into smaller, more intimate discussions, whereupon the woman turned to John and said gently, "John, you look very yin." She pronounced the word as "yeen."

John was taken aback and managed to say, "What do you mean?"

"You look yin—you know, passive, weak, like you've been eating too much sugar, candy, pastries, and stuff," she said. "You've heard of yin and yang, haven't you?"

"I've heard of yin," John replied. "Not yeen; I've never heard of 'yong,' pronouncing yang as the woman had. "What is it?"

Trying to drop a hint without lecturing him, the woman told John that he might be interested in the books of Michio Kushi or George Ohsawa. She mentioned a couple, then changed the subject.

The conversation once again resumed the energy of a bouncing ball, but the little words that had been bounced off John's mind had left an indelible impression.

A few days later, he telephoned the woman and asked for the titles of the books she had mentioned. She obliged, and he was off to the bookstore as soon as he hung up the phone.

There was a problem. John was down to his last $14.50, but he had an overpowering need to buy a macrobiotic book. Perhaps he could get one cheaply, he thought as he walked down the subway steps and took the train to an uptown bookstore.

At the store, John asked the clerk if he had *The Book of Judgment*, by George Ohsawa. No, said the clerk.

Did he have any books about macrobiotics? John asked. Yes, one. It was called *Macrobiotic Way of Life*, by Michio Kushi. Remarkably, the book was on sale—$10.95, down from $15.95. John smiled to himself and thought of his many friends "on the other side." He paid the man and headed toward the subway with just enough money to make it home by train. What luck! he thought—the book and a ride home. He held his new treasure as if it had been sent directly from above.

CHAPTER

6

I t was one of those rare evenings in the spring of 1983 when Michio and Aveline Kushi could spend some time at home together watching television. Michio had a news program on that featured several clergy members representing several religions talking about the AIDS epidemic. Michio had been counseling an increasing number of people with AIDS and watched the program with considerable interest. He could hardly believe what he was hearing.

The ministers and priests were uncharacteristically united: the AIDS plague, they said, was the wrath of God visited upon homosexuals. Homosexuality was a sin; those who engaged in it were therefore damned. AIDS was a kind of retribution visited upon gays and a warning to the rest of the human race to avoid homosexual behavior.

As he watched the program, Michio became angry. What a narrow view of life these men had, he thought to himself. They see AIDS as a single disease, confined to one small group of people, yet the causes of AIDS are everywhere in society, even among those who consider themselves righteous. What insight does their morality offer except to divide people into the good and the bad? Such thinking inevitably leads to war.

Michio's worldview could not have been more in contrast

with that of the clergymen. Rather than seeing people in terms of good and evil, his outlook was to regard all humanity as struggling to achieve balance in life, some people managing more successfully than others, but everyone suffering the consequences or reaping the rewards of that struggle.

The AIDS epidemic, in his view, was not the result of a small group of people behaving sinfully, but the natural consequence of an entire society out of balance with the Order of the Universe.

Michio had seen the destruction of human health coming for decades. He had traced the cycles of individual and social health throughout history, but the modern health crisis was clearly in evidence at the early part of the twentieth century. At that time, major changes in the Western diet began to take place. Between 1900 and 1970 consumption of whole grains, vegetables, and fruits was cut in half, from 40 percent in 1900 to 20 percent in 1970. Meanwhile, consumption of meat, butter, milk, and eggs rose. As a result, fat and cholesterol intake increased dramatically. At the turn of the century, only 30 percent of the average American's total calories came from fat, and much of that came from vegetable sources. By the 1970s, the total fat content of the diet hit 45 to 50 percent, most of it from animal foods.

At the same time, sugar consumption skyrocketed. By the 1970s, the typical American each year consumed 125 pounds of sugar. Soft drink consumption doubled between 1960 and 1975, with the average American consuming 295 twelve-ounce cans of soda pop in 1975. Sugar was also added to a wide variety of canned and packaged foods, including vegetables and condiments.

With the twentieth century came the widespread practice of refining grain. Whole-grain breads and flours gave way to white bread and white flour. Refining meant loss of important nutrients, especially minerals and fiber. Some of these lost nutrients were reintroduced by a process called "fortification," but refining still meant a net loss of nutrition.

Meanwhile, the use of chemical additives, including artificial preservatives, flavors, and colors became widespread. By the mid-1970s, there were 1,300 chemical food additives approved by the Food and Drug Administration for use in the American food supply. Some of these additives were proven to be carcinogenic, but no one could predict the subtle or long-term health effects of these chemicals.

Before long, the American diet consisted of great quantities of fat, cholesterol, sugar, refined grains, and chemical additives. Very few of these foods resembled those humans had grown accustomed to eating during their long evolution on the planet. Thus, the dramatic change in diet was an altogether unprecedented event in human history, a remarkable experiment that was causing changes in human biology that few people appreciated.

As the diet changed, the disease patterns of the West also changed, especially in the United States. In 1900, heart disease was the number-four killer disease among Americans, ranking well behind the number-one cause of death, pneumonia, and influenza. That year, heart disease killed approximately 10 people in every 10,000; influenza and pneumonia took 20 lives in every 10,000. Cancer was the number-eight killer in 1900, taking the lives of only 6 people in every 10,000.

By 1977, those figures had changed dramatically. Heart disease was now the number-one cause of death in the United States, taking 30 lives out of every 10,000—even more than pneumonia and influenza in their heyday—while cancer was the number-two killer, taking 17 lives in every 10,000. By the mid-1970s, heart disease was killing 1 million Americans annually, while cancer killed more than 400,000 each year, with 700,000 new cases of cancer being diagnosed annually. At the same time, 11 million Americans suffered from diabetes, 37 million from high blood pressure, and another 32 million from arthritis. The numbers were staggering. Degenerative diseases—especially heart disease and cancer—represented the greatest plague in the history of the human race.

In 1971, President Richard Nixon declared "war on cancer," launching a multibillion-dollar cancer research industry, but fifteen years later researchers conceded that little progress had been made in the search for a cure.

Finally, the 1980s saw a turn toward prevention of disease, which was less expensive and offered far more promise than the search for a cure. The focus on prevention was slow in coming, largely because preventive health methods were being championed not by doctors and scientists, but by laypeople.

By 1976, the U.S. Senate Select Commitee on Nutrition and Human Needs—led by Senator George McGovern—revealed that six of the ten leading causes of death in the United States were directly related to the American diet. The committee's report, called *Dietary Goals for the United States*, began an avalanche of diet-and-health information that was eagerly embraced by laypeople around the country. The health book trade reached annual revenues of $500 million, while newspapers, magazines, radio programs, and television shows regularly brought diet and health information to a public hungry for both. In 1979, the U.S. Surgeon General confirmed the findings of *Dietary Goals* and published *The Surgeon General's Report on Health Promotion and Disease Prevention*. The report recommended that Americans consume fewer meats, dairy products, and eggs and eat more whole grains, fresh vegetables, beans, fish, and fruit. Like *Dietary Goals*, the *Surgeon General's Report* stated that most degenerative diseases—especially heart disease and cancer—were caused largely by the typical American diet and life-style. Other reports followed, most notably the National Research Council's *Diet, Nutrition, and Cancer* (1982), which stated that fat consumption was a direct cause of the most common cancers, those of the breast, prostate, and colon.

There were even deeper problems, in Michio's view, that had to do with the way people thought about their eating habits and their health. The medical establishment relied almost entirely on two methods of treatment: drugs and surgery. The healing effects of diet and the body's own capacities to heal itself were dismissed or thought of as dangerously irresponsible.

Indeed, the pharmaceutical industry, with its plethora of pills and potions, had thoroughly convinced the average American that he or she could not live without a steady supply of aspirin, cold and cough medicines, birth control pills, and Val-

THE WAY OF HOPE

ium. Such medication created a nation of addicts, dependent upon pharmaceuticals for every sniffle, headache, or problem life presented.

Drugs fostered the attitude that the human body was the enemy, to be chemically manipulated into behaving properly. It also promoted the attitude that one could abuse one's body with food and drink, indulge in cavalier sex, or avoid the real issues of life with impunity. The solution was as close as one's medicine or liquor cabinet. And thanks to the advertising firms on Madison Avenue, it was all made to look so innocent. If one overate or drank too much the night before, one simply popped a couple of Alka-Seltzers or Bayer aspirins, and voilà, the pain was gone. What could be easier?

But it was precisely that kind of thinking that made Americans the perfect society for widespread drug addiction. For many it was but a short jump from over-the-counter medications to recreational drugs or alcohol abuse.

To Michio, it was a prescription for self-destruction.

Nature, in Michio's view, was constantly seeking balance between cause and effect. If one ate or drank too much, the natural consequences were upset stomach, heartburn, or diarrhea. This was balance. There was a lesson implicit in the experience that kept people alive and healthy: avoid certain foods and your digestion will work properly. Small violations of balance resulted in small consequences—diarrhea and colds, for example. By observing these simple laws, humans survived on the planet. But modern society had learned to indulge in harmful foods and alcohol and at the same time circumvent the consequences. Such a feat was made possible by drugs. Prescription and over-the-counter medication postponed the effects of harmful foods until the accumulation of toxins had become severe, thus resulting in equally severe side effects— heart attack, cancer, or a greatly impaired immune system.

Drugs didn't deal with the underlying cause of the problem; they dealt with the symptoms. They helped people avoid the causes of their problems, thus preventing anyone from effecting a true cure.

Thus the question of morality seemed irrelevant to Michio, or at least arbitrarily applied, since it was obvious to him that if blame were to be put on anyone, it would have to be applied to all of modern society, since virtually everyone was indulging to varying degrees in the same mistakes. The homosexual community, it was true, was currently bearing the brunt of the epidemic, largely because the life a great many of them had lived was so extremely out of balance, but for the most part the gay community had merely taken the existing mistakes to their natural limits. In other words, gays had reached an extreme point of dissipation more quickly than the rest of society.

Now, as Michio watched television, he turned to Aveline and said, "I'm going to New York to see people with AIDS."

Aveline thought for a moment and said, "Yes, I want to go, too."

The next day, he and Aveline made a plan to visit hospital administrators in Massachusetts and other nearby New England states to see if they could persuade doctors to set aside a limited number of beds so that AIDS patients could receive macrobiotic food while they were being treated medically. The Kushis would provide the food and the cooks.

Michio and Aveline thought it was a good idea, especially since the Lemiel Shattuck Hospital in Boston already had a successful macrobiotic food program. Each day macrobiotic foods were served to the hospital staff and to patients who requested the food. The program had begun in 1980 and had remained popular among hospital staff members.

In addition to the Shattuck food program, numerous studies of the macrobiotic diet had been done by Harvard University scientists, all of them confirming the positive effects of the diet, particularly those affecting cardiovascular health.

A few days later, Aveline set off on her prearranged appointments with hospital administrators. She brought along her oldest son, Lawrence (also known by his middle name, Haruo), who had recently obtained a doctorate from the Harvard School of Public Health. Lawrence was an epidemiologist and research scientist in the areas of nutrition and health. He not only possessed a deep understanding of macrobiotics, but also knew the science of nutrition and the great volume of research examining the link between diet and health.

Aveline and Lawrence's first stop was at a hospital in western Massachusetts. The Kushis have a home and macrobiotic school in Becket, Massachusetts, located in the Berkshires. It would be a good idea, they believed, if the hospital were located close enough to Becket so that the Kushis and certain senior students could supervise the program. The first hospital they visited was in western Massachusetts, near the New York State line.

Aveline and Lawrence arrived for their first appointment with the hospital administrator, who greeted them graciously. The Kushis explained that they wanted to set up a macrobiotic program within a hospital, to allow sick people access to macrobiotic foods, if they desired, and to monitor their health to see if the diet aided them in their recoveries. Aveline mentioned the Shattuck Hospital operation, which Larry explained in some detail. The administrator responded optimistically to the idea. He questioned Aveline and Larry regarding the additional supplies the hospital might need, and he discovered they were minimal. The hospital could even provide the food. In all likelihood, it would cost less than the existing diet, since meat, eggs, butter, and milk were more costly than grain and vegetables. Larry specified that the stoves would have to be gas, not electric. It is the view of macrobiotics followers that gas ranges cook food more thoroughly and more healthfully, that the gas flame is easier to regulate, and, in any event, that food cooked on a gas flame tastes better. No problem, the administrator said. The hospital used gas, but if there were not enough stoves in the kitchen, another could be added.

All was going well in the conversation. The CEO saw several potential benefits of having the macrobiotic program, not least of which was the public relations payoffs. He could probably envision the captions in professional journals already: "Massachusetts hospital experiments with vegetarian diet in the hope of speeding recovery of patients and reducing costs." Yes, it wouldn't be a bad idea at all.

Then Larry let the cat out of the bag, so to speak. Aveline and Michio wanted the hospital to allow patients with AIDS to eat the food. The Kushis had a special interest in AIDS because they believed the macrobiotic diet could help fight the disease. Would the CEO have any trouble with this? Lawrence asked.

The bright smile on the CEO's face vanished. AIDS was an entirely different matter. The disease was frightening; nobody liked dealing with AIDS patients, especially with their blood. There was a growing reluctance on the part of doctors to treat them at all; a minority of doctors had already announced their refusal to do so. There was also the terrible problem of public perception. People were afraid of receiving and giving blood. The community might panic if a special AIDS facility were established at the hospital. The CEO probably envisioned the headlines: "Massachusetts hospital experiments with vegetarian diet to treat AIDS patients." No, that wouldn't do at all.

A special program for AIDS patients would ruin the hospital's reputation in the community, the CEO explained. He hoped that the Kushis would understand. They did.

The answer was the same everywhere else. The Kushis met with other administrators, but each meeting had the same result. Hospital administrators were afraid of everything about AIDS: maintaining highly expensive facilities to handle the blood, dealing with hospital staff, and handling the public relations dilemma.

After they had become convinced that no hospital would help them, Michio and Aveline turned to religious organizations with connections to health care clinics or convalescent homes, but every time they were turned down. It was obvious that AIDS was not like other diseases; it gave rise to a special kind of fear.

By May of 1983, Michio and Aveline had given up looking for medical assistance and decided instead to go directly to the gay community. They realized, however, that they needed help. They couldn't just call up one of the gay community organizations because they were concerned that their efforts would be misinterpreted as taking advantage of the AIDS epidemic. What the Kushis needed was someone prominent and trustworthy within the gay community, someone who could act as a liaison between the macrobiotic people and gay organizations attempting to help those suffering from AIDS.

That spring Michio started making calls to macrobiotic friends in New York. One of the people he called was Kezia Schulberg, a young teacher of macrobiotic cooking in Manhattan. Michio informed her of his plan and asked if she would keep it in mind should the right person come along. She would.

That May, John Angelo was busy ruining every macrobiotic meal he attempted. But this night was going to be different, he told himself. This night he was going to Kezia Schulberg's house for a pot-luck macrobiotic dinner, where real macrobiotic cooks would prepare delicious, healthful meals. He had deliberately abstained from eating too much that day so that he could fully enjoy himself at dinner. When he arrived at Kezia Schulberg's apartment that evening, he was ravenous.

The food had been placed in serving bowls on the kitchen table. There were about a dozen other people at the house; John didn't know any of them. He introduced himself to Kezia and after a short conversation began to help himself to the food. He spooned large portions of brown rice, assorted greens, and beans onto his plate. He also took a small portion of hijiki seaweed, which didn't look half-bad. There were some sliced carrots mixed in the hijiki, and John detected the faint smell of lemon as he placed it on his plate and took a seat in the living room.

He had taken several bites before he finally decided that the meal was a disaster. The rice was hard, the beans and greens tasteless. The seaweed, however, wasn't bad—in fact, he enjoyed it more than any other dish. It was obvious to him that the food had been prepared by different cooks, but only one of them knew what he or she was doing. Surely, John thought to himself as he lifted some rice toward his mouth, the food could be made to taste better than this.

He ate enough to fill his stomach and then went over to meet Kezia, who immediately asked him how he had become involved with macrobiotics. John explained that he had been diagnosed with Kaposi's sarcoma and in all probability had AIDS. He was hoping that the diet could help him. He asked Kezia what she thought.

She was optimistic about his chances of recovery. "Have you read *Recalled By Life?*" she asked him.

"No," John said. "I just bought this one book by Michio Kushi, *The Macrobiotic Way*."

Kezia escorted him to the bookshelf in her living room and handed him a hardcover edition of *Recalled By Life*. "This is the book you should read," she said, handing him the book. He took it and read the dust jacket.

"May I borrow it?" he asked.

Kezia balked for a minute. She wasn't sure she wanted to part with it but relented after John, sensing her apprehension, assured her that he would treat it as if it were gold and return it within a week. Kezia agreed.

"By the way," John said, "is this good macrobiotic food?" He gestured to the plate in the lap of a young woman sitting nearby.

Kezia moved closer to John as if she were about to share a secret. "Oh, no," she said. "This is just terrible. All these people here are new; there isn't a single cook among them."

"Good," said John. "There's still hope." He and Kezia laughed and then he bade her good-bye.

That night, John consumed *Recalled By Life* as if it had been a gourmet meal. "It was a tangible manifestation of the principles Michio had written about in *The Macrobiotic Way*," he would say years later. "It showed me that despite all the doubts and the foreignness of the diet, it could be done by anyone who applied himself. And it could work."

The next few days saw an improvement in John's life. Since giving up his drug habit, he'd felt good about himself. He was following the diet as strictly as he could manage and feeling hopeful and positive. A few days after seeing Kezia, he sold two paintings and used part of the money to hire a macrobiotic cook. The cook came to his apartment five evenings a week for a month. Suddenly the food was delicious. John observed the mastery of the chef and took notes on everything he did. Now he followed the diet religiously, and there were immediate improvements.

"Within a couple of weeks, my energy levels improved dramatically," John recalled. "I felt lighter, stronger, happier. And I really believed it could help me."

Meanwhile, Oscar Molini and Michael Arlington were making miraculous progress. Late that spring, Michael's blood tests revealed a normal lymphocyte count, an event virtually unheard of in the treatment of AIDS. Oscar's blood test also showed a steady increase in lymphocyte count. His original blood test in July 1982 had indicated a count of 900 lymphocytes per cubic millimeter of blood; normal ranges from 1500 to 3500 cmm. But by the spring of 1983, Oscar's blood tests were showing that his lymphocyte count was well into the 2000-cmm range.

His doctor was more than surprised. He declared that Oscar was undergoing some sort of miracle. Meanwhile, Oscar was trying to tell his physician that his improvement was due to his dietary habits, a point of view the doctor politely declined to accept.

Nevertheless, despite his doctor's incredulity, Oscar was convinced that the diet was working and, more important, that he was well on his way to recovery.

Meanwhile, many of Oscar's friends were dying.

The losses were having a terrible impact on Michael. That spring he decided that he could no longer bear New York. The strain of the city and the spread of AIDS had affected his relationship with Oscar as well. The two were arguing more now. Finally Michael decided he had to get out of the city. Late that May he moved to Atlanta, where he had lived before moving to New York five years earlier.

There was a growing panic among Oscar's friends, as one after another received the terrible diagnosis from physicians. Bill Shulman was one such friend. He had been diagnosed with

AIDS earlier that year, but recently he had dropped from sight. Oscar telephoned him periodically, but the phone just rang without an answer. Concerned, Oscar phoned other friends and asked about Shulman's whereabouts. No one seemed to know.

Bill had a couple of treasured pet parakeets in a giant wooden cage in his living room. Every time he went on vacation or spent a few days away from his apartment, he took great pains to see that the birds were well cared for. It was an inside joke with his friends—neurotic Bill and his pampered birds. After a while, people started to wonder who was the real captive pet, Bill or the parakeets.

"Who's taking care of Bill's birds?" Oscar kept asking friends. But no one seemed to know.

When several weeks passed without any word from Bill, Oscar finally called Bill's landlord and asked if he'd seen Bill.

The landlord was irritated with Oscar's call. "They took him away," he said as if the whole world had already been informed.

"What happened?" Oscar asked urgently.

"The ambulance took him away. He let the birds out of the cage, they were flying all over the place. He went crazy. He was under the table yelling at the birds."

"Where did they take him?" Oscar asked.

"Lenox Hill Hospital," replied the landlord.

Oscar rushed to Lenox Hill Hospital and located a nurse who was familiar with Bill's case. "What happened to him?" he asked.

"He's got AIDS," the nurse said.

"I know," said Oscar. "But why was he hospitalized so suddenly?"

"He contracted spinal meningitis. It spread to his brain. He became delirious."

"Can I see him?" Oscar asked.

"Yes, but he's been heavily medicated; I think he's sleeping," said the nurse. "And you'll have to wear a mask. He's very contagious."

Oscar went into Bill's room. Bill lay in bed, looking at the ceiling. He was emaciated, a skeleton with skin. The colors of his skin varied with the contours of his skull, running from slightly blue to pink to brown. His eyes, nose, and lips all seemed to be reaching out, looking to communicate with something invisible. The expression on his face suggested that he was suffocating, but after looking at the rise and fall of his chest, Oscar noted that he was breathing normally. The whole story was in Bill's eyes. They bulged and remained unblinking as if they bore witness to a demon so hideous and malicious that they had to remain fixed on it, lest by looking away the thing might escape.

Oscar went to his bedside and said, "Bill, it's Oscar."

Bill didn't seem to notice Oscar, but the sound of his voice triggered a response. Bill started babbling incoherently. He was making lists, telling himself to remember to do things. "Get the groceries, return the library books, get bird food, feed the birds, let the birds out, let the birds out . . ." On and on he rambled. Bill was still talking to himself when Oscar left the room, shattered.

Oscar trembled all the way home. Something terrible had happened. Bill wasn't even recognizable—that wasn't Bill, that was some delirious soul waiting to die.

Why am I getting better while my friends are dying? he kept asking himself. Why isn't that me? Will it be me?

Oscar had been telling his friends what he was doing to help himself against the disease, but most of them treated his adopting macrobiotics as evidence of his desperation. He felt helpless and tortured. He wanted to do something for Bill, but seeing him like that frightened Oscar to the point of panic.

When he got home, he called Cheryl and told her about Bill. She was tough and to the point. "You have to think about saving yourself now, Oscar," she said. "I think you should stay away from hospitals until you have fully recovered and have the strength to deal with sick people. Until then, your main priority has to be yourself. Get better and then you can do something for others. You're no good to others or to yourself if you're dead."

It sounded harsh and even a bit cruel, but Oscar knew in his heart that Cheryl was right. He had to minimize the losses for the time being.

Oscar felt all the more alone now. Not a week passed, it seemed, that he didn't hear of some old friend or acquaintance being diagnosed with AIDS. Over the next five years, he would lose more than thirty friends to AIDS. Meanwhile, other friends who didn't contract the illness were constantly telling him of their own losses, either longtime friends or lovers who had been destroyed by the disease. AIDS dominated everyone's consciousness. It was just below the surface of every conversation. Sooner or later the subject would come up; everyone would become fearful and then morbid. Such talk became little more than a roll call of death.

In July Oscar felt he needed more than dietary guidance; he needed spiritual nurturance. Cheryl recognized the problem and asked Oscar if he would join her for a special gathering of friends who were welcoming May Li Loa Shin, a Buddhist teacher from Hong Kong whom Cheryl had known for many years. May Li was about to arrive in New York after teaching in Austria.

May Li was no ordinary woman; she was regarded by Cheryl and thousands of students around the world as a Buddhist master who was not only a teacher of religion but a highly evolved human being possessed of rare insight. Oscar had never heard of her but agreed to join Cheryl and some of her friends at a macrobiotic restaurant in New York to meet May Li. The minute May Li entered the restaurant, Oscar was happy he had decided to accept Cheryl's invitation.

May Li was English, with a fine, angular face, accented by her large blue eyes and patrician nose. Her age was difficult to gauge; she might have been in her mid-forties, but Oscar couldn't be sure. Her hair was brown, long and straight with no trace of gray. She was tall, thin, and moved with a confident bearing. She had a look in her eyes of certainty, yet playfulness. She wasn't stuffy, but she seemed sure.

About a dozen people were present at the adjoining tables; it was too large a group to get into serious conversation, so Cheryl suggested to Oscar that a smaller group get together with May Li that night at Oscar's apartment. Oscar was game.

Forty-five minutes later May Li and six others, including

Oscar, were sitting in his living room talking. Suddenly May Li turned to Oscar and asked him why he thought he was living. Oscar was taken aback. "I don't know," he said. May Li's steady gaze rested on him, waiting for an answer.

"Why am I here?" Oscar said, repeating the question. "I never really asked that question of myself before."

"What do you want to become?" May Li asked.

"I don't know," Oscar replied. "I guess I want to become a successful artist and businessman, to be appreciated by my fellow workers, to leave my mark."

"That's rubbish," May Li said without any attempt to soften her words. "That's what you think you want, but you don't even know what you want."

Oscar felt as if he had been punched in the nose. He became withdrawn for a few minutes while the emotional fireworks went off inside him. Meanwhile, others began asking questions and May Li answered, but Oscar was so overwhelmed by the encounter that he couldn't follow the conversation.

Suddenly the night was over and May Li was leaving. Oscar, seeing everyone to the door, overheard Cheryl inviting May Li back to Oscar's apartment the following night for another session. Oscar heard himself say that that would be wonderful, but he was mildly disoriented and couldn't be sure of what he was saying.

The following day, Oscar invited six of his friends to sit with May Li and share ideas. Two were militant gay activists; the others were suffering from AIDS. The six friends had expected May Li to be there around 7:30 P.M., but they had to wait until 10:30 for her to arrive with Cheryl and two other women in tow.

The two gay activists were already upset at having been kept waiting. They were combative and wasted no time going on the attack with questions about May Li's views on homosexuality and AIDS.

What followed was a kind of intellectual judo. The seven gay men, including Oscar, were thrown around the room, while May Li never raised her voice or worked up a sweat.

May Li asked them what they wanted. One man said he wanted liberation.

"The spirit is always free," May Li said. "That's what you really are. You're not this homosexual ego. You are something much more important than your sexuality. You are a human spirit.

"You're putting youself into this small cup and saying you want liberation. You put a label on yourself and then get angry and fight for liberation. But you imprison yourself. You've made being gay the most important thing in life, and now it's your prison. You go around saying I'm this, you're that, we can't communicate. So you go to the people who accept you and reinforce your thinking.

"AIDS is not the result of being homosexual, it's the result of your life-style, which is your ego. Your life-style is a denial of the spirit. How can such a thing bring about health?"

The activist charged back. "We've worked so hard for liberation," he said. "We've made important gains, changed minds, changed society."

"Liberate yourselves from a life that is totally materialistic, sensorial, and destructive. Then you'll be free," said May Li.

May Li left that night and the following day returned to Hong Kong. But her words ripped open a door in Oscar that had been slightly ajar since he had begun macrobiotics. He was both galvanized and confused. He didn't know what he was going to do next, but he felt changes coming on him like thunder on the horizon. The ground on which he had built his personality was shaking.

In late July he decided he could not remain in New York; it represented too many of the wrong things to him now. He wanted to go home. He returned to Miami and took up residence with his parents for a while until he found his own place.

That summer John Angelo went to Kezia's house regularly for meals and assistance with the diet. The two became close friends. One night in July, Kezia told John that Michio Kushi was coming to New York to give a lecture on diet and health and to do some personal counseling. "Perhaps you could meet him," Kezia suggested.

John was taken aback. Meet Michio Kushi? he thought. Maybe in five years, after I've practiced really well and I know something about what I'm doing.

"I don't think I can afford a consultation with him," John told Kezia.

"Maybe you could just meet and ask him a question about how you're doing," Kezia said.

"No. I couldn't do that," said John. "I hate people who try to rip off others by using some personal contact to get free advice."

Kezia didn't push it but asked John to be there to help her with the appointments. He agreed.

Michio arrived that August and gave a public lecture at the Intercontinental Hotel in Manhattan on diet and health. He talked briefly about AIDS. Later, he gave private counseling sessions in one of the conference rooms of the hotel suite. Outside, Kezia kept track of the appointments, shepherding people in to see Michio and answering questions afterward. A few hundred people had attended Michio's lecture, and many wanted to see him privately.

Midway through the appointments, Kezia came over to John and said that Michio would like to talk to him. Excited and surprised, John went into the conference room and sat down on a chair opposite Michio. At Michio's right was Bill Spear, a longtime student of Michio's and senior macrobiotic teacher.

"How are you?" Michio asked with a smile.

"I'm fine," John said.

At this point, Bill Spear broke in. "No, Michio means, 'How are you doing on the diet?' "

Now John was uncomfortable. He didn't want to act as if he were soliciting free advice, but he wanted to ask a thousand questions. "No problems," he said.

"Are you doing all right with the cooking?" Michio asked. "Are you enjoying the food?"

Now it finally hit John that Michio was trying to draw him

out; he wanted John to ask any questions he might have. But John kept the reins on himself; he kept thinking, I don't want a free ride. He also thought about the large group of people waiting to see Michio and the collective trauma they represented. He didn't want to take too much time. But he felt something else, too.

"It was obvious that right then Michio's only concern was me. It was just he and I, human to human," John recalled. "He radiated friendship and caring, and I could have sat there all day. I was so excited to meet him, but I didn't know what to say."

Finally he said: "I'm enjoying the food and I'm not having any trouble following the diet."

"Good," Michio said in a long, low breath, the smile never leaving his face. "You are doing very well. I wonder if you could act as a liaison between my office and the gay community? We would like to see more friends with AIDS who want to begin macrobiotics."

John was even more surprised now by Michio's request. "I don't think I'd be very good at that," he said. "I just started the diet myself, and I don't know a whole lot about macrobiotics."

"You'll be very good," said Michio. "Will you do it?"

John said, "Yes, if you think it will help."

Michio smiled and said thank you—John was just the man he was looking for.

CHAPTER

7

On June 28, 1969, Jim Fouratt, political activist, actor, and gay man, was walking down Christopher Street in Greenwich Village when he spotted police running into the Stonewall Inn, a bar and nightclub that was well known as a popular club for gay men. The police raided the bar and closed it on a liquor license violation. But as they tried to empty the Stonewall, some of the men inside refused to leave. Angry words were exchanged. Nightsticks were wielded. Fists began to fly. Suddenly a riot broke out. Thirteen people were arrested, four policemen were reported hurt. For the first time, the gay men at the Stonewall had openly resisted the police and, by extension, a society they claimed had oppressed them for too long. It was a turning point. Gay liberation was born.

For three days—June 28, June 29, and July 3—demonstrations and riots took place at Sheridan Square in Greenwich Village protesting the raid on the Stonewall and claiming that the police had now become the official instrument of society's homophobia, or its fear and hatred of homosexuals. Five hundred demonstrators gathered at Sheridan Square on June 29. Fighting broke out between demonstrators and police, with three people reportedly arrested. On July 3 a new demonstration formed at the square with more violence and more arrests.

Jim Fouratt was among the leaders of the demonstrations. For him the protests were an extension of the activism he had already been engaged in as a leader against the Vietnam War. Fouratt was one of the founders of the National Liberation Front, a leftist organization committed to seeing an end to the war. Still, Fouratt and many others believed the movement to end the war was only part of an ongoing human revolution that, it was hoped, would transform American society forever. As far as Fouratt was concerned, the confrontation between the straight and gay communities was long overdue.

After the Stonewall riots, Fouratt and a few of his friends created a new group, which they called the Gay Liberation Front.

The Gay Liberation Front was concerned not only with the liberation of gays from the hatred and discrimination of the heterosexual world, but with the larger question of human freedom in society. As the leadership of the Gay Liberation Front saw it, human sexual preferences were the inherent right of each individual. Society didn't have the right to dictate sexual orientation to any one of its members, as long as the individual did no harm to others. To be subjected to violence or discrimination or to be ostracized from the community because of one's sexual choices was nothing less than a deprivation of basic human freedoms.

The Gay Liberation Front organized demonstrations for equal rights in cities across the country. It called repeatedly for an end to discrimination against gays, created Gay Pride Weeks in New York and other major cities, and in general gave homosexuals a platform from which to speak out against what they saw as society's institutionalized homophobia.

Remarkably, gay liberation gained momentum and power almost overnight. Meanwhile, other gay organizations were formed, including Gay Activist Alliance. Leaders of the movement became increasingly outspoken and politically active, with various organizations backing political candidates and forcing politicians to address the issues facing homosexuals.

To be sure, gay liberation had a great deal of help. The sexual revolution of the 1970s and the women's rights movement brought about unprecedented change in sexual roles and attitudes.

According to Fouratt and other gay leaders, however, gay liberation turned away from its more general goals of human revolution to one exclusively focused on sex. The need for sexual freedom was somehow transformed into a movement for abundant sex, which itself became a way of expressing one's freedom and realizing a political anthem. Like a giant moon that eclipsed the sun, sex obscured the more important goal of love. And that, Fouratt would later say, led inexorably to AIDS.

Many gay leaders began promoting promiscuity as a political statement. It was a rebellious act, a thumbing of the nose to the straights who deemed such behavior scandalous, sinful, despicable. Having sex was, in itself, a refusal to accept the morality—and thus the values—of the straight world. But there were consequences. Having promiscuous sex led invariably to disease.

"A lot of gay men developed the consciousness that being gay meant just two things: having a lot of sex and being sick all the time," said Jim Fouratt. "The problem was that this definition of being gay obscured the person's humanness, so that sex eclipsed all other aspects of their lives. They became sexual beings, not human beings."

From the shadow of gay liberation came a new industry: commercial sex. Bathhouses, sex clubs, paraphernalia, and drugs became the basis of an enormous industry within the gay community, providing not only the related services of sex, but jobs, advertising in newspapers and magazines, support for other businesses, such as printing—in short, the basis of a community economy.

"Some people made enormous fortunes selling poppers [amyl nitrate]," said Fouratt. "It was white, middle-class gay men who were selling the drugs to other gays. It was gay men who owned and operated the bathhouses, sex clubs, and encouraged drug use and promiscuity."

Gay entrepreneurs took full advantage of the new openness and the demand for abundant sex.

One of the remarkable events of the decade was that the entire gay economy was allowed to proliferate without serious antagonism from law enforcement officials. Any number of laws were being broken every day, not least of which was prostitution and drug peddling.

Without any real restraint from the law, or any serious critique from within the gay community itself—many of the newspapers and magazines were themselves dependent upon the advertising from sex-related businesses—the gay community was about to suffer the consequences of too much success.

In June 1981 five homosexual men in Los Angeles were diagnosed with rare cases of pneumonia called pneumocystis carinii pneumonia (PCP). The disease, which is caused by a common airborne parasite, is easily destroyed by a well-functioning immune system. But these men were unable to overcome the parasite because their immune systems were no longer functioning. The five cases were reported to the CDC in Atlanta. A month later twenty-six more gay men in New York and California were reported to be suffering from this rare disease state in which their immune systems had completely shut down. Slow but steady reports of this same disease began to surface, most of them from New York City, San Francisco, and Los Angeles. All the cases involved gay men. Most of the men contracted either pneumonia or Kaposi's sarcoma, a cancer that normally afflicts older people who are able to survive indefinitely with the illness. Unlike these cases, however, the gay men with Kaposi's were dying rapidly. Finally, in July of 1982, several hemophiliacs contracted this immune deficiency syndrome after receiving blood supplied from hospitals in major metropolitan centers.

By 1982 the number of cases of AIDS was still small, about five thousand, but the disease was spreading rapidly. Also, it appeared to be confined, at least initially, to the gay community and to a tiny percentage of people receiving blood donations. The effect of AIDS upon gays and gay liberation was devastating. Before AIDS, gay men faced the specter of syphilis, gonorrhea, and amoebic dysentery, all of which could be taken care of by drugs. Now they faced death. Moreover, the rise of AIDS resurrected the ugly message gays had fought against so long and hard: that the real disease was homosexuality.

In many ways the 1970s had been good to Jim Fouratt. He emerged from the war years having dealt extensively with his homosexuality and the conflicts that his sexual preferences engendered in him. He did not engage in promiscuous sex as so many of his brethren did. Instead he maintained long-lasting relationships with friends and a lasting love relationship with one man.

To be sure, he had his problems, including addiction to alcohol and amphetamines. Of his own volition, Jim entered a 12 step program that helped him give up drugs and alcohol. He remained in the program for nine years; meanwhile, he underwent psychotherapy and confronted his demons directly. Jim Fouratt emerged with a rare degree of integration and balance.

His business life went well, too. Fouratt had become a major nightclub owner in New York and was now among the movers and shakers in the city's club and dance scene. In 1979 he took over a small dying disco called Hurrah in lower Manhattan, brought in live music—mostly New Wave and punk—and turned it into a success second only to Studio 54. In 1980 he opened a second club called Pravda in the Soho district of Manhattan, which provided a cabaret atmosphere, live performances, and music. It, too, became a hit. Fouratt then started a string of new clubs, including Danceteria and the Peppermint Lounge, all of which experienced almost overnight success. With his background as a political activist and modest success as an actor— he had studied with Lee Strasberg at the Actor's Studio for seven years and performed on Broadway and television—Fouratt was well known in New York among the beautiful people who frequented his nightclubs and who counted him among their friends.

But then, in 1981, one of Fouratt's best friends was stricken with AIDS. The friend died a slow, horrible death, with Fouratt at his bedside. Just before his friend finally let go, Fouratt made him a promise.

"I promised him that I would take a year and try to find an answer," Fouratt recalled.

He took time from his businesses and began his promised search. His first step was a descent into the hell that is AIDS.

That hell afflicted everyone in the gay community, the healthy and the sick. To some extent, gays were always dealing with the inherent dualism of their circumstances—the mentality of "us versus them," "gay versus straight." But now a strange new dichotomy had split the gay community: the sick versus the healthy. Gays were suspicious of one another; doubt now divided friends and lovers. If love within the gay community was hard to come by before AIDS, it was downright rare immediately after it.

"A generalized terror gripped the gay community," Fouratt recalled. "Doctors didn't offer the slightest hope. There was nothing they could do except to make death a little easier." But death was inevitable.

The kind of death offered by physicians had to be considered as well. The principal methods of treatment for most AIDS patients at the time were chemotherapy and Interleukin 2, the latter drug representing the only hope physicians had of stimulating the immune system in the face of AIDS. Neither one promised a cure, and both had devastating side effects.

"There are definitely circumstances when medical intervention is needed, and that includes chemotherapy," said Fouratt, "but what we had to do was weigh the pros and cons and see if the chances of success with certain highly toxic remedies were really warranted. Chemotherapy can be devastating; it can strip a person of his dignity before it kills him. Death is never pleasant. But it's even worse to be chemically tortured and then die."

Meanwhile, evangelists and moralists seized upon the obvious public relations aspects of the disease. A great deal was made of divine retribution. References to Sodom and Gomorrah as biblical metaphors for the current age became clichés.

Self-hatred surfaced with a vengeance. The utter hopelessness engendered by the disease gave it deep psychological and even spiritual implications. The evidence was powerful in itself: the medical profession's utter failure to find an answer combined perfectly with the moralist's doctrine of divine retribution. Together, the doctor and the evangelist brought new life to an old idea that homosexuals were cosmically cursed, that here was a disease beyond medical science and, more important, beyond forgiveness.

In the early part of 1982, Fouratt formed one of the first support groups for people with AIDS called Wipe Out AIDS. The group was composed of twenty people then, most of them men with AIDS, but a small number of them healthy men and women who wanted to help AIDS patients.

One of the healthy members of the group, a man named Sid, told Fouratt that his lover had just been diagnosed with AIDS.

"What are you going to do about it?" Jim asked.

"I don't know," said Sid. "Everyone is telling me to leave him, but I really don't want to. I don't know what to do."

"It sounds like he needs you now," Jim said.

"I know," said Sid. "But everyone is telling me that if I stay with him I'll die, too."

"Do you think it's right for us to be abandoning those we love when they need us most?" Jim asked.

"But what about me? If I stay, I'm at risk."

"That's true, but only if you are not careful with sex," said Jim. "There's more to love than reckless sex."

Sid stayed with his lover, a man named Paul. Together, they attended the Wipe Out AIDS meetings and began practicing the methods of the 12 step program Jim Fouratt fostered each week.

The ground rules of the meetings were simple. First, everyone had to develop the ability to listen.

"Listening is a real skill," said Fouratt. "You have to feel that you can share your experience with others who are receptive and uncritical. That's very important. It provides both the speaker and the listener with perspective; the one who's talking feels relieved of the pressure, and those who are listening recognize that they are not alone in their fear. Being able to listen to another person is a powerful healing tool, because it communicates that you care, that you respect the person you're listening to. That's love."

Fouratt discovered that simply providing a safe place for people to talk reduced the fear they were experiencing.

"Allowing people to express their fears enables them to externalize them and look at them with some degree of objectivity," said Fouratt. "Then they can begin to deal with fear more effectively."

The big fear, of course, was death. "The first thing we have to acknowledge is that each of us is going to die," said Fouratt. "In the 12 Step Program, you have to take responsibility for the time you have. You must take the active role in living. That means that each day you do what you can to further your life and your goals, and then you turn it over to a higher power. That higher power is different for each person—some refer to it as God, others as Tao, whatever, but you have to recognize that you can only do so much and then you have to turn it over to some other higher power to do the rest. You do the best you can and then you let the results be."

The effect of such an attitude was, in Fouratt's experience, transforming. "People began to relax. They didn't have to do it all. That was liberating because each of us secretly knows that we can't do it all.

"We take life one day at a time. We do what we can do. And the quality of life is much different because now the person is actively living, not simply waiting to die."

One of the great obstacles Fouratt and his group faced was the overwhelming sense of powerlessness that gripped those afflicted with AIDS. That powerlessness emerged from the idea that gays were victims of AIDS, and that the illness had struck randomly. Such thinking was even fostered among many gay men because it served a purpose: it allowed people to maintain the delusion that they were innocent of the causes of AIDS. But as far as Fouratt was concerned, there was a dangerous other-side to such thinking: it promoted the notion that once afflicted with AIDS, there was nothing anyone could do to affect the disease or the quality of life one experienced. In other words, people were choosing to be powerless because it satisfied other needs, especially those involving self-image.

But the notion of innocence and powerlessness did not improve the chances of recovery or the quality of life. As un-pleasant as it sounded, those afflicted with AIDS had to take responsibility for their conditions if they were ever to find a way of solving the problem or living decent, responsible lives for whatever time remained.

"We started to look at self-hatred and the sources of self-hatred, which was a kind of internalized homophobia," Fouratt said. "When society tells you all your life that you are sick and hates you for your sexual preferences, you start to believe that there is something wrong with you and then you begin to hate yourself. And that self-hatred becomes the basis for self-annihilation."

Many gay men discovered that self-hatred infused their identity as homosexuals. It prevented them from looking for loving relationships because they believed they didn't deserve them. As one of the men in the group put it:

"For years I visited the bathhouses and bars and had sex with a lot of men, but what I was really doing was substituting sex for intimacy and love. I thought I couldn't have real love, I wasn't good enough, so I got the next best thing, which was sex. And I got a lot of it."

When self-hatred becomes acute, death is the only salvation.

"One of the early recognitions we all had," said Fouratt, "was that down deep many of the men who contracted AIDS really believed that they deserved to die." AIDS facilitated that death wish perfectly. The only answer to such a death wish was to bring some sort of balance to self-hatred—which, of course, is self-love.

"Learning to love yourself is no easy matter—not for anybody—but for gay men it can often begin with the realization that human beings are more than their sexuality," Fouratt said. "When you realize that, you can begin to look at other parts of yourself and see things that are worth nurturing in yourself, things that you like about yourself, that really deserve your love. You can see yourself in balance, and I think that is the beginning of self-love."

The support group clearly had a positive effect on both Sid and Paul, who, despite his diagnosis of AIDS and Kaposi's sarcoma, remained relatively symptom-free for the next six years. He had bouts of fatigue, periods of weakness, and night sweats, but he continued to survive despite the fact that he used no medical or alternative therapy. (Paul is still alive in 1988, six years after diagnosis.)

Despite the psychological and spiritual victories, Wipe Out AIDS still suffered heavy losses. One of Jim's closest friends, a Broadway actor, contracted the disease and died the most horrible death Fouratt could ever have imagined. The young man literally turned green, his fingernails and toenails clubbed, his whole body seemed to shrivel up and writhe in pain.

It was also clear that the group needed more than what was being offered by the medical establishment or by the psychological and spiritual approaches it was currently employing. Thus, Wipe Out AIDS launched a search into alternative therapies being offered. The organization was particularly concerned about the quality of the approach and its cost, especially since AIDS patients were so susceptible to quacks and charlatans.

"We looked into everything that was being offered at the time—megavitamin therapy, herbs and supplements, chiropractic, various home remedies, including many of the drugs being peddled. Some of the members experimented with this therapy and that one. We also invited alternative healers to our meetings to listen to their ideas about health and specifically about AIDS."

In August 1983, in the midst of this search for answers, one of the members brought to the group's weekly meeting a flyer that advertised an upcoming lecture on AIDS by Michio Kushi. The title of the lecture was "The Cause and Recovery of AIDS." Fouratt was intrigued. "Let's go to this," he said to the members. "Let's hear what Michio Kushi has to say."

CHAPTER

8

The large lecture hall at the Intercontinental Hotel was filled with about two hundred people. Jim Fouratt and several of the members of Wipe Out AIDS sat a few rows from the front. Fouratt wanted to get a close look at Michio. Like others in the audience, he was suspicious. Nearly fifteen years before—in the late 1960s—Fouratt had practiced macrobiotics for a time. To be sure, it was his own brand of macrobiotics: brown rice, seaweed, pickles, and amphetamines. He believed in the philosophy, though. The whole idea of balance appealed to him. The notion that food was directly related to health and that good health enhanced other aspects of life were vague ideals, but compatible with Jim's philosophy.

But then he began to read the macrobiotic literature more deeply and uncovered some rather incompatible—if not downright repulsive—elements in George Ohsawa's writings. Ohsawa had argued that homosexuality was a sickness that could be cured by appropriate diet. Ohsawa maintained that yin and yang took human form as woman and man. Since yin and yang were complementary opposites—both incomplete without the other—it was only natural that man and woman should be attracted to each other and ultimately unite for the creation of new life. That a man might be sexually attracted to another man—or a woman to a woman—was for Ohsawa a violation of the Order of the Universe.

It wasn't just that Ohsawa regarded homosexuality as a sickness; the way he wrote about it left little room for discussion. He often saw things in black and white.

But for Jim Fouratt and many others, Ohsawa's inflexibility on the subject of homosexuality was too much to bear. More homophobia, Fouratt thought. He dropped macrobiotics and forgot about the more appealing aspects of the practice, lumping the whole thing together under the rubric of heterosexual prejudice.

Fouratt had never met Michio Kushi but suspected that the yin-yang dialectic had led him to conclusions similar to those of Ohsawa, particularly with regard to homosexuality.

Michio himself had written that diet was implicated in the choice of sexual direction one took in life, but he tended to be nonjudgmental in such matters. It was a choice, he said, which diet facilitated or helped to bring about, and he left it at that. Later, when he would be questioned at length by the gay community of New York, Michio would state his feelings in no uncertain terms.

Jim Fouratt shifted anxiously on his chair waiting for the lecture to begin. Despite his concerns about homophobia, he was eager to hear what Michio had to say about AIDS. He was ready to listen to anyone.

The past year and a half had been a long walk through hell. There had been so much suffering, so much death. The tragedy of AIDS hung on the gay community like heavy shackles, imprisoning each person in fear. Fouratt could feel the collective sadness and hopelessness of those present. The depression seemed almost palpable, as if it were an entity unto itself. He turned around on his chair and scanned the crowd. How strange it was, how terribly foreign, to see so many familiar faces that had previously radiated such daring and courage, sensuality and intimacy, now reflecting only fear and paranoia. AIDS was war without hope of victory. He could see defeat in the slumped postures of the audience and the suspicion with which people greeted one another, especially friends they hadn't seen in a while. The spirit was dying before the flesh.

Yes, Fouratt was ready to listen, but he was poised to strike if necessary. He was prepared to take Michio to task at the first sign of homophobia or the first mention of an unfounded or dangerous claim. War eliminated any room for loose talk.

Finally Michio appeared at the back of the room and walked to the podium in front of a blackboard. He placed a short piece of paper on the podium in front of him and then walked in front of the lectern and stood before his audience. He spoke in his simple English, shaped by his strong Japanese accent.

"Each year, one million Americans die of heart and artery diseases," he said. "Nearly forty million Americans suffer from cardiovascular disease. Five hundred thousand people will die of cancer, and another one million will be diagnosed with cancer this year. Eleven million suffer from diabetes. Nearly three hundred thousand Americans suffer from arthritis. The list of illnesses goes on and on. And each year, the numbers get higher and higher. Each year, more and more people suffer from chronic degenerative diseases.

"When I was a boy," Michio said, "we never heard of cancer. No one knew what this disease was. Heart disease? No one had heart disease. Then, gradually, more and more people became sick. Today, every family knows someone who has cancer or who has died of cancer. Everyone knows what cancer is.

"Now, AIDS. This is the greatest threat to the health of the world. It will spread very rapidly. By the year 2000, many millions will suffer from AIDS. It will affect all parts of society: government leaders, doctors, scientists, artists, business people, the average man and woman. Everyone will know someone who has AIDS.

"Heart disease, cancer, diabetes, arthritis, now AIDS—humanity is getting weaker. More and more people getting sick. Immune system is getting weaker. People are more susceptible to disease.

"As a result, more medicine, more surgery, are needed to keep people alive and functioning every day.

"In the past sixty years, the diet has changed very much.

"In the morning, people eat what? Eggs, which have plenty of fat and cholesterol; bacon, also plenty of fat; butter, also fat. Or, they have a doughnut, which has plenty of sugar. At about ten o'clock in the morning, they feel weak, tired, depressed. They have low blood sugar. What do they want? A Snickers bar, or some other candy. Another doughnut, maybe. Lunchtime comes, people eat bologna sandwich, roast beef sandwich, hamburger, hotdog—all fat and cholesterol on white bread. Between meals, people eat plenty of candy, ice cream. Dinnertime comes: people hurry to McDonald's, Wendy's, Burger King. Or they have TV dinner, or they cook steaks, roast beef, potatoes or French fries, a little frozen vegetables. After dinner, more snacks, ice cream, cake, candy. The whole diet is fat, sugar, white flour, and chemicals.

"What do you think this eating does to people? It makes them weak. They become weaker and weaker.

"Then people get sick. What do they do? Right away, they take aspirin, other medicines, antibiotics, and painkillers. The body wants poisons from diet to come out. But people don't want to suffer the consequences of their day-to-day eating, so they take drugs to stop eliminations. The drugs make symptoms go away, but underlying problem is still there. Only gets worse. More medicine is needed. More Pepto-Bismol, Tums, cold medicines, antibiotics. Soon, stronger medicine is needed. Heart is troubled; angina pain is coming all the time. Or a lump comes out on skin, or in breast, or some other place on body. Doctor has to cut it out. Maybe he has to take out organs, too. Intestines have to go out, spleen out, sex organs out, breast taken off. Arteries around heart have to be replaced. Electronic pacemaker put in heart.

"But the way of eating day to day, the way of life day to day, this is the real problem. If the diet is not changed, if lifestyle is not changed, then the problems just get worse. If you treat only the symptoms, the disease gets worse."

Michio turned to the blackboard and drew a tree with long roots into the soil. He made many tiny dots to indicate germs infecting the tree.

"The tree is sick," he said. "Let us say that the germs have not destroyed the power of metabolism in tree, but just caused sickness. What do we do for the tree to make it well? If we just spray chemicals on tree, then germs inside will not go away. The way to cure the tree is to improve soil and water. That will make the tree stronger. When tree is stronger, germs go away. The tree becomes inhospitable to the germs. This is the tree's immune system working.

"Same approach is necessary against disease, including AIDS. Change the nutrition of a person, his daily food and drink, and he will become stronger. Natural immunity will become strong again.

"Suppose we use chemicals to treat AIDS. All drugs have side effects. Sometimes drugs are so strong that they have a poisonous effect. They weaken immunity, so death comes quicker. Sometimes that death is very painful.

"If we do not change our approach, the underlying cause of the disease will never be addressed and the disease will continue to spread. If we do not make ourselves stronger, make natural immunity stronger, we are in danger of losing the human race.

"In five years from now, more than three hundred thousand cases of AIDS will be in this country alone. Millions will be carrying AIDS virus. In Africa, many more millions will have AIDS. By this disease alone, whole population can die out."

Here, Michio paused. He seemed to be thinking of something. The silence in the room was loud; it had the effect of drawing the audience closer to him.

"What is cause of AIDS?" he asked. "Let's look.

"I have seen and talked to many people with AIDS. Every AIDS person I have seen eats plenty of sweets: sugar, chocolate, candy, honey, plenty of desserts. They also eat plenty of fat from dairy foods, like cheeses, milk, butter, yogurt, cream, and ice cream."

Michio gestured as if he were spooning ice cream into his mouth. "Plenty of banana splits, with chocolate ice cream and cherry on top—so good," he says, laughing. A ripple of laughter ran through the audience.

"They eat lots of fruit juices, and fruits, especially tropical fruits. They don't eat so much meat—just a little bit, mostly chicken, fish—but sometimes hotdogs and hamburgers, but less meat than sweets.

"Then, they take plenty of drugs: cocaine, LSD, marijuana, sleeping pills, diet pills, antibiotics.

"We say that sweets, creamy dairy foods, sugar, tropical fruits, and fruit juices are very yin. These foods are very soothing and delicious. They create expansion; they loosen and cause decay in the body. These foods cause the body to lose minerals. The body loses minerals, so bones and teeth decay, muscles become weak. Too much yin. Too much fatty foods and sugar.

"Natural immunity needs minerals to be strong. But sugar robs immune system of minerals, making it weak.

"Also, this yin diet is very rich in fat, especially saturated fat from dairy products, like cheese, milk, milk shakes, and ice cream, and from fast foods, like hamburgers and hotdogs. Fat weakens immunity. Fat coats immune cells, like macrophage and helper T cells, so that they lose sensitivity and cannot respond to the presence of disease. Also, fat and sugar together create an acid-rich environment in the bloodstream, which is hospitable to virus, germs, and bacteria. Disease flourishes in blood that is rich in acid.

"Naturally, people who eat this way every day get weaker and weaker. When they encounter disease, they cannot fight it off because immunity is weak.

"In addition, they take plenty of drugs which suppress immune response and makes immunity even weaker, so that it cannot fight disease.

"Finally, they have plenty of sex partners. Sperm goes into their bodies from many different people who have many different health conditions. White blood cells attack this sperm because it is foreign to the body; also, very often it is not healthy sperm—illness comes with it. Many AIDS friends have had many sexually transmitted diseases, such as syphilis, gonorrhea, amoebic dysentery. Also, many have suffered from liver diseases, like hepatitis. These diseases stay in the bloodstream. The immune system must fight them every day, day after day. This weakens immunity, too.

"Then, AIDS comes. People become sick. But the problem was there long before AIDS came.

"Whole human race now suffering from this pattern. Everyone eating plenty of fat and sugar. Everyone trying to achieve comfort. People eating plenty of fast foods, ice cream, soda pop, taking plenty of drugs. That means that health of whole human race is going down.

"AIDS is not so-called gay disease. It is disease that all of humanity must deal with.

"What can we do? Should we wait for cure? Should we wait for vaccine? Maybe vaccine or cure will be here in ten years or so, maybe not. Maybe, like cancer, cure will not come for generations. What can we do? Whole human race is threatened. This is big problem.

"To understand cause and cure of AIDS, we must understand life. Life is balance. Sickness is imbalance.

"Cause of AIDS is yin. Too much expansion, too much acid in bloodstream."

Once again Michio turned to the blackboard. This time he drew a man on the board, then turned his attention back to the audience.

"We say yin is expansive. Therefore, yin foods cause energy in body to move upward and to the periphery. Yin causes face to become red; pimples come out; hands become red at knuckles and joints. Capillaries in skin of face and hands become swollen.

"Meanwhile, strong acid in intestines causes diarrhea, intestinal infections. Intestines become perfect host for microorganisms—bacteria, amoebas.

"Blood is cleansed by liver, by kidneys. When bacteria and infection gets in blood, liver must clean it; infection goes to liver. Blood is filled with fat, cholesterol, sugar, bacteria, acid; liver becomes overwhelmed. Liver cannot eliminate infection from the body, so disease is stored in liver. Organs that clean blood become infested with disease themselves.

"Lymph becomes burdened. Lymph is like garbage man for body, trying every day to clean blood and take out bacteria, foreign matter, but lymph becomes overworked and swollen with too much garbage. Lymph nodes become swollen. Pollution of body is building and building; cannot eliminate it. More and more, it is stored in lymph, in liver, in kidneys, blood.

"This is perfect environment for disease. Blood becomes more acid-rich. Bacteria thrives. Germs spread. Intestines have parasites. Then sickness comes. AIDS.

"With AIDS people, very often they get Kaposi's sarcoma— cancer with lesions on the skin. This is yin discharge. Cancer is on the surface of body, at the periphery. Very rarely will cancer be found in young AIDS friends deep in body. Always, it is on the surface. Kaposi's is yin.

"For people with AIDS, the cause was too much yin. Too much expansive foods, chemicals, and life-style that included excessive amount of sex and too many sexual partners. All of this is expansion.

"Too much yin makes very emotional person. Too much yin makes chaotic behavior. Can't control behavior. Can't make order in life. Whole life becomes too expanded, disorderly, and chaotic.

"What is the answer? What can we do?

"When there is too much expansion, balance comes by creating contraction. Contraction is yang.

"The cure for AIDS is to make balance with yin condition. For that, we need more yang foods and yang, orderly behavior. This is only way to restore immunity.

"How do we do it?

"We begin with good diet. Every day, eating well.

"For that, we use macrobiotic diet."

Again Michio turned his attention to the blackboard, and on the left side, where there wasn't anything drawn or written on as yet, he drew a circle and a pie diagram within it to indicate the percentage of each food the men should eat.

"Fifty to sixty percent of diet each day should be whole cereal grains, such as brown rice, millet, barley, steel-cut oats, and buckwheat. Twenty to thirty percent should be vegetables, natural, organic vegetables. Mineral content is high in organic vegetables and they have no pesticides. Also, vegetables are rich in fiber. Five to ten percent beans, including aduki beans, lentils, chick-peas, navy beans, pinto, black beans, soybeans, and tofu and tempeh. Every day, small amounts of sea vegetables, such as hijiki, nori, arame, kombu, and wakame seaweeds. Sea vegetables are very rich in minerals. Every day, soups, such as miso soup and tamari broth. Very easy to make, very delicious soups. Then, small amount of fish is okay, but white fish that is low in fat, such as flounder, cod, and haddock. Sometimes, if you crave sweet taste, a small amount of cooked fruit is okay, but small amounts, and only when you crave sweet.

"We have to be careful with extremes of both yin and yang, because too much yin makes us crave strong yang, and too much yang makes us crave strong yin. We are looking for balance."

Here again, Michio paused to collect himself and the audience.

"We can't say whether we can cure AIDS. No one can say that, because no one has proven it yet. But we can improve our health. Even if we are sick now, we can improve. No one can say how much we can improve our health. That is up to you. Many can overcome AIDS. Those who eat well and maintain a healthy way of life can live long, and be healthy. This I know to be true."

With that, Michio turned to two people sitting in the front row of the audience and motioned for them to stand up. "I would like you to meet a couple of my friends," he said, calling them to him at the front of the room. He gestured for them to turn to the audience, then introduced them as John Angelo and Richard Medrano. "Please, tell them your story," he said. John and Richard took turns telling the audience their experiences.

Richard Medrano was a thirty-year-old free-lance design artist specializing in prints, fabric art, wall hangings, and window displays for some of the more fashionable department stores and boutiques in Manhattan. Soft-spoken and refined, Richard was a Mexican American who had come to New York nearly a decade before. He was about five feet seven inches tall, with a small, handsome face and black crew-cut hair that seemed to balance nicely against his fine clothes.

Richard had a steady lover, but he frequented the baths and the bars and engaged in casual sex routinely. He also did the so-called designer drugs that provided the on-demand euphoria so much a part of the elegant circles he moved in. In the fall of 1982, Richard was diagnosed as having AIDS and Kaposi's sarcoma. Shortly thereafter a friend introduced him to macrobiotics; he also told Richard about a macrobiotic cook in Greenwich Village by the name of Billy Kohler, who had been macrobiotic for some ten years and ran a cooking school out of his home. Richard got Billy to cook regular meals for him and to begin teaching him how to cook.

Richard was religious about his diet. His transgressions were macrobiotic desserts. Beyond that, he adhered strictly to the letter and spirit of the law. He told the audience that in the months he had been following the diet, he had observed many improvements in his health, especially a dramatic increase in energy, a loss of excess weight, and a deep feeling of vitality and strength. The Kaposi lesions had not gone away; he hadn't had another blood test, he said, but he presumed that his blood levels were essentially the same as they had been at diagnosis. Still, he was feeling better. It was a vague but promising sign. Certainly he wasn't in the hospital dying. He was hopeful that he would overcome his disease.

When it was all over, Jim Fouratt was overwhelmed. "Michio was the first person I had encountered who provided some hope. I was so moved by him, by his spirit and caring, I can't tell you." John Angelo's "story was very inspirational as well. I decided then that macrobiotics was really worth looking at."

Two weeks later Fouratt contacted Michio and arranged a

date in November for him to address a gathering organized by Fouratt and Wipe Out AIDS, to take place at the Lesbian and Gay Community Center in Greenwich Village. In the meantime, Fouratt got in touch with John and Richard, both of whom quickly became active members of Wipe Out AIDS.

The group welcomed them both with open arms. Wipe Out AIDS was desperate for direction and hope. John and Richard were the embodiments of both.

The facade of the Lesbian and Gay Community Center on West 13th Street in Manhattan is the color of dirty blood. It is an eerie, iron-red building stained with pollution. Fencing covers the windows to protect it from break-ins; the paint is chipped and peeling, and some of the windows are so covered over with soot as to be impervious to light.

The interior is even more depressing. A small lobby leads into a large, cavernous room. In November 1983 the walls were the color of army fatigues, olive drab. Uncovered light bulbs, yellowed with dust, hung from chains, shedding a weak light into the room. The white pillars supporting the ceiling cast long, diffuse shadows. The ceiling was tin, also painted white but badly rusted. The green-and-black linoleum-tiled floor was dulled by ground-in dirt. Posters, pamphlets, and papers advertising workshops and political gatherings—many of them for safe drugs rallies or seminars on homosexual life-styles—littered the bulletin boards, walls, halls, and rooms. Entering the Lesbian and Gay Community Center meant stepping into another world, a world reminiscent of old B movies in which the characters play out some low-intensity drama, like a slow-moving dream, in shades of black and white.

The building itself is 155 years old. Before becoming the Lesbian and Gay Community Center, it served as a butchery and baking school. Although it had been abandoned for years, the gay community was able to secure it only after long delays and considerable red tape, which was interpreted by many gays as the city's attempt at keeping the building from the homosexual community.

Jim Fouratt and the members of Wipe Out AIDS rented the building for Michio's lecture. Gene Fedorko, an old friend of Fouratt's and a recent member of the group, had advertised the meeting throughout the five boroughs.

Among the hundred people waiting for Michio was Gary Marks, a thirty-seven-year-old accountant who had been diagnosed with AIDS and Kaposi's sarcoma in September. The diagnosis had not come as a complete surprise to him.

Gary had a long history of sickness, and there had been many premature deaths in his family. His mother's family had been decimated early in life: her sister had died at birth; her brother had been killed in World War II; and her own mother had herself eventually died in childbirth. Gary grew up in Brooklyn, New York, listening to stories of death. He recalled the times he would come into the kitchen and find his mother standing alone at the sink crying about the loss of her brother and mother.

Gary was very close to his older cousin, a woman who had served as a surrogate mother to him. In 1956, when Gary was ten, his cousin died suddenly of a cerebral hemorrhage. Her death confirmed all his darkest suspicions and convinced him that it was only a matter of time before death caught up with him, too. At the age of ten, he was close to having a nervous breakdown. His doctor prescribed children's liquid Thorazine, a tranquilizer, which he took for months.

But from that point on, Gary was a hypochondriac. He suffered from allergies, perpetually swollen glands, chronic colds, and a host of psychosomatic symptoms. He was constantly being taken to his doctor, who prescribed penicillin and other antibiotics. His medication became his crutch, the only thing that gave him any sort of security. The very presence of his medicine seemed to serve as a buttress against death, as well as a reminder of how close it was.

As compensation for his many troubles, his parents allowed him to indulge his cravings for sweets and ice cream. Gary ate a pint of ice cream a day; it was routine in his house to make sure he had his ice cream every night.

Naturally, Gary suffered from low self-esteem. In addition to being weaker than the other kids, he looked like Howdy Doody. Unfortunately for him, his sister looked like Grace Kelly. Gary's parents liked to compare the two, with Gary usually getting the unfavorable comments.

There was another problem, one as disturbing as death. He had strange feelings around other boys, an almost unbearable attraction. He was only twelve years old when he first began to notice these feelings. At first he didn't realize that he was different, but he was becoming aware that the other boys didn't feel the same way. Obviously, he must keep his feelings secret. His secret troubled him greatly, and as the years went by the trouble only grew worse. Finally, when he was about fifteen years old, he went to the public library and surreptitiously searched the racks for anything that might give him some insight into his secret. After considerable effort, he found a book. It was small and yellowed with age, almost hidden among other books that were written on the mysterious subject of sex; the others, however, were not concerned with his particular secret. He paged through the book and noticed continual references to the word *homosexuality*, which described the secret accurately. However, the fact that it was the only book on the subject and that it was so slim didn't reassure him. The book seemed like a secret itself. He left the library that day wondering if he weren't afflicted with some strange disease.

As time passed his difference was more apparent. He didn't like sports; he liked art. But his parents and teachers steered him away from what he liked—further evidence of his deviance, he decided. His attraction to other boys continued. The other boys, however, were clearly attracted to girls. Gary spent his teenage years in alienation. Like that little book in the library, he was alone and lonely, too small to be important, too big and far too different to disappear.

At the age of twenty he moved to Manhattan, finished business school, and found the homosexual ghetto. It was a revelation. "I discovered that there were other people like me," he would say many years later. In fact, in Manhattan there were quite a number of people who called themselves "gay."

The cork had finally come off the bottle; the genie was allowed out. Gary spent the next seventeen years leading a double life. During the day he climbed in the business world and at night he partied in gay discos and bars. Over the years a funny thing happened. His looks changed. "By the age of thirty-two, I was gorgeous," he said later. This homely little Jewish outsider, who had been whispered about and ostracized, was suddenly desired by many gay men. And Gary reveled in the attention and indulged in the sex as if it were ice cream. He went wild. It wasn't unusual for him to have sex with up to twenty men a week.

Despite the fact that he was physically attractive, he was filled with self-criticism and self-hatred. He could be bitingly critical of others as well, focusing outward the contempt he felt within.

"Even after I got to New York and started being desirable, I still had low self-esteem," he recalled. "I was using sex as a substitute for love. But I didn't even think of love then; I never thought I deserved it, and I didn't think I'd ever get anyone to really love me. Sex was the only thing I ever really expected."

Gary continued to take antibiotics and other medications as if they were staples. On the other hand, he was deathly afraid of recreational drugs and avoided them entirely.

Remarkably, Gary was in psychotherapy for twenty-two years, beginning when he was a teenager. But it altered neither his life-style nor his fundamental attitudes about himself. About the only thing his psychiatrist was good for was regular prescriptions of Valium, which Gary took in moderation whenever he faced a stressful situation, such as a plane ride or an important business meeting. Valium was his support.

In 1981 Gary read an article about AIDS. This illness is going to get me, he said to himself. Two years later, on his way home from a vacation in Israel, he discovered a strange sore behind his ear. He immediately contacted his physician, who, after taking a biopsy of the lesion and running a series of blood tests, informed Gary that he had AIDS and Kaposi's. The prognosis was that he had approximately two years to live.

Gary had had a distant acquaintance with Oscar Molini. He knew that Oscar had AIDS and Kaposi's; he also knew that he was practicing macrobiotics as a therapy for the disease. Then, in late October, he saw one of the Wipe Out AIDS posters for Michio's lecture.

Now he waited for Michio to arrive, eager to hear something that might give him reason to hope. Others, including John Angelo and Richard Medrano, cherished that same hope.

Right on cue, at seven-thirty, the Kushis arrived, and Michio mounted a small dais that had been constructed for him between two pillars to speak to the three hundred men and women assembled. (One of the men who attended the lecture would later liken Michio to a skinny version of Samson, standing between the pillars, about to bring down so many misconceptions about life and about AIDS.) Aveline sat on a free chair in back of the room.

Aveline had not been to any of the lectures to the gay community before. Now, as she scanned this grim room and saw the terrible sickness and misery on the faces of these young men, she had all she could do to hold back the tears.

"I had such a bad feeling," she said years later. "These people were like green grass, still young, but starting to die. The building was old and dirty and not well cared for. The whole feeling was depressed. I didn't think this would work out," she said. "I didn't think we could do anything for them, then."

Now, more than ever before, Michio saw what AIDS was doing to the gay community. He felt the weight of depression and surrender in the people he stood before. The oppressive atmosphere of this building and the absence of hope on the faces of those present, made him realize that most of these people were simply waiting to die.

He tried desperately to uplift them. He peppered his presentation with jokes, especially about the common addiction to sugar, ice cream, and other dairy foods that afflicted those he called "AIDS friends."

"We have so many friends here tonight who came straight from Baskin-Robbins," he said. And it was true. Several men sitting in the audience were spooning ice cream into their mouths as Michio spoke. They knew nothing of the macrobiotic diet or its philosophy. They had come because they had seen a poster with "AIDS" on it. But now the ice cream caused some embarrassment.

"Today, people want comfort. Prosperity means comfort," Michio began. "People want convenience; they do not want difficulties.

"Prosperity can make people weak. The average American now is fifteen pounds overweight. Difficulties make people stronger; tolerance is immunity.

"Today's diet is not for health but for convenience. Modern people want to eat fast food, have tasty food without much cooking. Everyone's very busy. On the go. Food has to be prepared fast; many people go to fast-food restaurants, like McDonald's, where the food has plenty of fat, salt, and sugar."

From here, Michio outlined the common dietary pattern of Western children.

"While mother is pregnant, she eats plenty of sweets, she drinks plenty of soft drinks. That means lots of sugar. Coca-Cola has plenty of caffeine, sugar, and chemicals. Meanwhile, mother eats lots of fat in the form of meat, dairy products, and eggs; she eats lots of white flour, in the form of white bread, rolls, and pastries. Mother may go to fast-food restaurants, eating French fries, hamburgers, milk shakes, Coca-Cola.

"Baby lives on mother's blood. So baby inside mother's womb is growing on this diet, which is very weakening. Baby is born very big, fat, and weak.

"So-called baby boomers, children born after World War Two and in the 1950s, these babies got plenty of sugar, refined foods, chemicals, and fat from mother's diet.

"When baby is born, what does mother give baby? Cow's milk. Whole generation of mothers in 1940s and 1950s were told that mother's milk is inferior to cow's milk.

"Breast milk makes child's immune system stronger for child's entire life. The first three days after baby is born, mother's milk is yellow. This yellow liquid is rich with immunity. Today, most young adults were not breast-fed as babies. Therefore, their immune systems are much weaker than those who were breast-fed.

"Child grows up and eats plenty of candy and dairy foods—sugar and fat; not so many vegetables. They eat no whole cereal grains. That means very little minerals, fiber; loss of many vitamins; they ate lots of fat and sugar.

"The lymph system cleans the blood. But poisons going into blood every day from daily eating. Lymph system becomes burdened. So lymph glands become swollen. This causes tonsils to become swollen and infected. Then doctor takes tonsils out. This operation is so common. No one thinks twice about it.

"Tonsils were not made so that doctors could take them out," said Michio. Here a wave of laughter ran through the audience. "Tonsils become swollen and infected for a reason.

"Something made tonsils become swollen. Operation doesn't change that underlying problem. But the loss of tonsils is a loss of immune function. Tonsils serve a purpose; they are part of the lymph system. The body doesn't have unnecessary parts. Now lymph system is weaker. Tonsils are missing.

"After tonsils come out, children eat what? Ice cream, plenty of ice cream. Ice cream is cold and filled with fat and sugar. Cold shocks stomach and intestines. Fat and sugar increases burden on lymph system.

"From time to time, child gets cold or becomes sick. Child may get fever. Fever is the body's way of making the internal environment unpleasant for virus or bacteria. Fever is actually the body's answer to disease. But right away, we give drugs to lower fever. Medicine prevents immune system from doing its job. Then doctor gives antibiotics.

" 'Anti' means against. 'Biotics' means life. 'Antibiotics' means against life. Antibiotics kill microorganisms in the intestines. Kill all life in intestines, don't discriminate. Many microorganisms are beneficial to digestion; they help the body get more nutrients from food. Antibiotics destroy them. As a result, we cannot get as much nutrition from the diet, and digestion becomes weaker.

"Intestinal environment becomes more unhealthy. Many unhealthy bacteria begin to live in intestines. Candida albicans—from yeast—comes, causing so-called candidiasis. This bacteria makes acid. Also, anaerobic bacteria comes, which consumes oxygen and gives off carbon dioxide in intestines. These bacteria thrive in fat-rich environment. These bacteria give off estrogens. Hormones become imbalanced. Estrogen fuels cancer cells.

"Also, in acid-rich intestinal tract, parasites can come and live very easily.

"Meanwhile, day-to-day eating is producing more acid in blood, intestines, and cells, making happy home for germs. More fat comes into blood and intestines and cells, causing more anaerobic bacteria to grow, making estrogens.

"All of this comes because we do not want to experience the results of our actions. We want to avoid the effects of what we do. But you cannot avoid consequences forever.

"Immune system is working all the time to fight the effects of the diet, drugs, behavior. This means immune system gets weaker and weaker.

"Then sex life is excessive. Many gay friends have many ejaculations. In one week, many friends are ejaculating twenty to thirty times. This means a great loss of energy. Semen is made from blood and proteins. The more ejaculations, the more the body must work to produce more sperm and semen. This is a tremendous loss of energy and nutrients, especially proteins. Many ejaculations each week, fifty-two weeks a year, year after year—this causes the body to become weaker and weaker.

"In order to conserve strength, you shouldn't ejaculate more than two times a week.

"Even worse, many friends are having sex with many partners. They take sperm into their bodies.

"We say that semen is very yin. It contains millions of sperm, which got out of body and move very quickly and cause great expansion, or growth. Woman produces one egg for fertilization. Woman is yang; she produces one egg, and keeps it within her body. This is yang, contraction. Woman's egg is yang. It is very compact little ball. It doesn't move much in comparison to sperm, which travels a great distance to reach egg. Sperm is yin; egg is yang. Therefore, they attract. Together they create new life.

"If man takes semen into his body, it makes him more yin, more weak. Also, immune system comes to fight this sperm, making immune system all the more tired and weak.

"Is this life-style promoting health? Of course not.

"People don't think about what affects their health. They think about what feels good right now. All of this means that we are looking for convenience and for sensory satisfaction.

"We are always looking for comfort, but too much comfort and convenience can make us weak. Comfort makes us less adaptable to the changing environment. Difficulties make us adaptable and strong. If humans can't adapt, they die out, like dinosaur."

From here, Michio outlined the standard macrobiotic diet and placed special emphasis on chewing each mouthful of food thirty-five to fifty times. He said that failure to chew food results in enormous stress on the intestines and more acidity in the stomach. He maintained that saliva is an alkalizing agent, and that the more one chews, the more saliva is mixed in the food, thus making the food easier to digest and assimilate.

After he finished outlining the diet and answering questions from the audience, Michio addressed himself to the issue of hope. Yes, there were many difficulties ahead in dealing with the problems of AIDS, but they were not insurmountable if we began now to improve our way of life, he said. Much could be done to restore the immune function and to lead healthy, happy, and rewarding lives.

"Day-to-day practice has to be very good. We can't cheat, but if it is good, there is hope. Let us begin together to overcome this problem and to recover our natural way of health and vitality.''

With that, he descended the dais, walked up to one of the men seated in the front row, and embraced him.

Following Michio's lecture, Wipe Out AIDS began to grow rapidly. Its macrobiotic orientation was now well established. The group contacted several senior macrobiotics consultants, including Bill Spear from Middletown, Connecticut; Denny Waxman from Philadelphia; and Murray Snyder from Baltimore. These three macrobiotics teachers made regular trips to New York to provide instructions in the macrobiotic way of life.

In addition to the guidance of the macrobiotics leadership, there was the support and advice of John Angelo and Richard Medrano, both of whom committed themselves to helping everyone and anyone who wanted to use macrobiotics as an adjunct treatment for AIDS. Meanwhile, Jim Fouratt and Gene Fedorko, who gradually emerged as a leader within Wipe Out AIDS, sought the counsel of other alternative healers, particularly those who emphasized the relationship between the mind and body. Guests were invited to meetings where they could share their thoughts on health, sickness, and AIDS in particular.

Gary Marks became a regular at such meetings. Immediately after Michio's lecture, he sought out Jim Fouratt and, with Fouratt's help, found a macrobiotic cook to begin preparing his meals.

Others joined the group. Among them was Max Pestalozzi DiCorcia, twenty-eight years old. Max was five feet nine, with short dark hair, big round eyes, and a soft-spoken, friendly manner that covered the intensity of a rage that burned just beneath the surface. Max was gentle toward others but violent toward himself. He was living then on Avenue B in lower Manhattan, a part of town famous for its flourishing drug trade, muggings, and stabbings. The drug business went on uninterrupted right below Max's apartment window twenty-four hours a day. On Sundays he watched as the cars lined up, nine deep, with license plates from New York, New Jersey, Pennsylvania, and Connecticut. You could get anything you wanted on Avenue B, and more than you could handle.

Max was proof of that. He was an IV drug user, mainlining mostly cocaine and heroin. He kept his habit going by street theft and burglaries. He was also promiscuous, visiting the baths and sex bars weekly, as well as picking up strangers on a regular basis.

In September of 1983, just two months before Michio's lecture, Max was diagnosed with AIDS and Kaposi's sarcoma. A month later he saw the Wipe Out AIDS poster and, after Michio's talk, began attending the group's meetings.

Almost miraculously, Max—a man who had grown accustomed to the underside of life—adopted the diet and life-style religiously. He attended cooking classes provided by Billy Kohler, who gave them at Richard Medrano's apartment. He also studied cooking himself and soon became quite adept at the art.

Meanwhile, the Kushis came to New York regularly to provide lectures, counseling, and cooking classes. In December of 1983, Aveline gave a cooking class at the home of Jackie Windsor, a macrobiotic woman who had a large loft in Greenwich Village.

About fifty people crowded into her large kitchen and dining area. Many of them had never been to any kind of cooking class before, much less one specializing in macrobiotic dishes.

Aveline was dressed stylishly in a black blouse and skirt covered by a flower-printed smock. Her long black hair was pulled straight back in a ponytail, and her soft eyes and large smile were radiant.

She showed them how to cook a standard macrobiotic meal of pressure-cooked brown rice, steamed greens and carrots, beans cooked in tamari soy sauce, and arame seaweed, with a garnish of sesame seeds and lemon juice. She explained every step she took in her simple English, from time to time asking her audience for help with a particular word. When she could not express herself in words, she spoke with her hands, making gentle spirals in the air or over a pot, or by making a slow, sweeping gesture upward to show how certain foods would create a more uplifting spirit in daily life. She laughed in a self-deprecating way about her troubles with the language or a meal she remembered burning.

The fifty people present represented a cross section of men obviously concerned about AIDS and women with a general interest in macrobiotic cooking.

About midway through the class, a young man stood up and announced that he had something to say. For a minute everyone froze in surprise because Aveline was in the middle of cooking and the man, who was about thirty years old, was obviously ill. He had recently undergone chemotherapy, and most of his hair had fallen out. Patches of short red hair had begun to grow back, but the effect of the new growth, in combination with the painful pallor of his skin, was to shroud him in the shadow of death. Everyone knew that he was gravely ill. Tension gripped the group; no one was sure what would happen next.

Aveline looked up at him and, tilting her head slightly, smiled in expectation.

Suddenly the young man began to cry. "No one has cared like you have," he began. "Everyone hates us. You're the only ones who have cared. I just want to thank you."

Now the tension was unbearable. The man sat back down, and Aveline, obviously moved by the young man's gratitude, nodded to him and said softly, "Thank you." Then she went back to stirring her beans.

Such gratitude these people have, Aveline thought to herself. I think there is still hope.

CHAPTER 10

I n the fall of 1983 there was little interest in the study of AIDS within the mainstream medical community. The prevailing view that this disease was isolated within the homosexual population kept grant money—the lifeblood of scientific research—running at a mere trickle.

For Elinor Levy, an immunologist and research scientist at Boston University, the problem was bigger than money. She wanted to study AIDS, but she could not locate a steady supply of AIDS-infected blood to use in her research. Most major research centers had not begun taking blood samples, and those that had—such as Mount Sinai in New York—didn't have blood in sufficient quantities to pass on to other scientists.

Elinor Levy had more than a casual interest in AIDS. She had graduated in 1963 from Brandeis University with a bachelor's degree in chemistry. In 1972 she received her doctorate in biophysics from Emory University and for three years did postdoctoral work in biophysics and immunology at the University of British Columbia at Vancouver. In 1975 she became a research associate at the Cancer Research Center at Boston University and then an assistant professor within the Department of Microbiology at BU. By 1984 Dr. Levy was an associate professor at Boston University, specializing in microbiology and the immune system. AIDS fell within her special field of expertise, and Levy wanted very much to make a contribution to the search for an answer. Yet despite her credentials, her interest, and the fact that she worked at a major university, Elinor Levy's hands were tied.

While she hunted for blood samples, a colleague at BU had an offbeat interest that would provide crucial assistance. Robert Lerman, M.D.-Ph.D., head of the Boston University Hospital, had been studying cancer and its link to diet. Lerman had read the account of Dr. Anthony Sattilaro's recovery from prostate cancer in *Recalled By Life* a year before and was trying to determine how many other people with cancer had had similar experiences on the macrobiotic diet. Lerman had met Lawrence Kushi when Kushi was a Ph.D. student at Harvard and was now working with Lawrence in trying to track down people who had used macrobiotics to treat cancer. In the course of their collaboration, Lawrence told Lerman about his father's work with AIDS patients. Lawrence said that his father was seeing a number of men in New York City who had an interest in using the macrobiotic diet to treat AIDS. In fact, Michio was now looking for some medical assistance to study the blood of men with AIDS who consistently practiced the macrobiotic diet. Lerman passed on the information to Dr. Levy.

Elinor was intrigued. She knew nothing of macrobiotics— she hadn't even heard of it before—but after talking to Lerman she saw the possible research benefits in collaborating with Michio Kushi. For one thing, AIDS-infected blood was usually polluted with drugs, thus making it more difficult to do accurate research. By themselves, drugs affected blood values and immune response. These factors obscured test results and prevented the scientist from isolating the specific effects AIDS had on white blood cells. It was already difficult to get samples of AIDS-infected blood, but to get it free of drugs was even tougher. Levy telephoned Lawrence Kushi, and the two agreed to meet.

In February 1984 Lawrence and Elinor Levy boarded a flight from Boston to New York to meet representatives from Wipe

Out AIDS at the Lesbian and Gay Community Center in Manhattan. It was early evening when they entered the old building and made their way through the paper-strewn hallways. Elinor noticed a poster that read "How Far Is Too Far?" At that moment, she watched as one woman led another through the halls by pulling on a chain leash that was wrapped around the second woman's neck. Elinor swallowed hard and made her way to the small office in the basement, where she met Jim Fouratt, Gene Fedorko, Robert Angelo, and other members of Wipe Out AIDS.

Lawrence and Elinor explained their plan. They would like to study the blood samples of men with AIDS who were following the macrobiotic diet. Elinor had a variety of tests she wanted to run on the blood samples but would regularly report back to the men on their immune parameters. The tests would cost them nothing. All they had to do was submit to testing consistently.

Fouratt, Fedorko, and Angelo liked the idea. They realized that they needed some type of medical intervention to see what effect, if any, the diet and life-style was having on the men. If macrobiotics was useless, the men could move on to other possible therapies. Elinor Levy represented a chance for concrete answers—something that would benefit everyone. Wipe Out AIDS was happy to cooperate.

Elinor explained that she would need a list of men who wanted to participate in the study and some basic medical information. She handed Fouratt a sheaf of forms; he promised to talk to the group and report back to her shortly.

Now the study could begin. But there was just one hitch: the group needed a medical doctor in New York who could take blood samples and monitor the health of the men. This was a crucial element. The person would have to be unique—he or she would need both a medical and scientific background and an appreciation and understanding of macrobiotics to help the men with their practice—an unusual combination of talents. Elinor and Lawrence discussed the problem on the way home to Boston. Lawrence said he had an idea.

*   *   *

Dr. Martha Cottrell sat in a coffee shop in midtown Manhattan and waited for Michio Kushi. She was eager to talk with him about the plan outlined on the telephone by Lawrence Kushi.

Martha had grown up in Alabama. She married at the age of sixteen, had three children, and then, at the age of twenty-five, entered Mercer University in Georgia. At the age of thirty Cottrell was accepted by Woman's Medical College in Philadelphia and graduated four years later in 1962. She began to practice in Long Island, N.Y., as a board-certified family practitioner. However, in the early 1970s she developed an interest in the connection between mind and body and began studying with Ilana Rubenfeld, a New York scientist and teacher of psychoneuroimmunology.

Through the 1970s Martha experienced acute arthritis pain in her shoulders and back, for which she could find no answer. The plethora of aspirin and prescription painkillers she took failed to cure the pain. Her condition only grew worse. She suffered from acute and recurrent sinusitis, with accompanying headaches. She developed gastroenteritis, or intestinal pain and swelling. Her personal frustrations with medicine were replicated in her medical practice; so often after she prescribed a drug, her patients were only temporarily relieved and eventually returned with the same problems, usually more severe. Most of the time drugs merely postponed the inevitable.

On July 3, 1978, Martha awoke with an acute case of inflammatory arthritis and arthritic psoriasis, a severe skin rash all over her body. Her joints, back, and shoulders were locked in pain. Her every move produced agony. When she finally managed to get herself to a local physician, she was told that she would need cortisone for the arthritis. Martha had resisted taking the drug for years. She had had cortisone injections for bursitis but no longer wanted to continue its use for fear of its numerous side effects, including hormonal imbalance, weakening of the immune system, more symptoms of arthritis, and increased susceptibility to illnesses such as diabetes and

Parkinson's disease. Cortisone was a last resort—once taken there was no turning back from it; cortisone either worked or didn't, and its failure could wreak havoc elsewhere in the system. Still unwilling to commit to the treatment, she decided to wait a little longer.

Martha had a physician friend who was interested in holistic medicine. He had suggested that she look into alternative treatments for her numerous illnesses, which she did. She began to read a wide variety of books on holistic health. She was particularly intrigued by the work of Dr. O. Carl Simonton, whose book *Getting Well Again* (J. P. Tarcher, 1978) had documented the effects of attitude on immune response. She also became interested in the work of Nathan Pritikin, who was effectively treating a wide variety of degenerative diseases, including heart disease, high blood pressure, and arthritis, with a diet of whole grains, vegetables, beans, and fruit.

Her study of holistic medicine continued. In 1979 she attended the annual meeting of the Holistic Medical Association in Wisconsin, where she met a wide variety of practitioners in the fields of nutrition, acupuncture, and psychosomatic medicine. In September 1980, after she read an article in the *Saturday Evening Post* about Dr. Anthony Sattilaro's recovery from cancer with the use of a macrobiotic diet, she bought several books by Michio Kushi and George Ohsawa and plunged into the study of diet and health and the philosophy of yin and yang.

Within days of reading the magazine article, Martha had decided to adopt a macrobiotic diet. She struggled with cookbooks, a whole new set of recipes, and most of all the foreign foods on the diet. Within six months she experienced a remission of arthritis pain and sinus headaches. Gradually her skin and intestinal disorder also cleared up. Her experience opened up a whole new world for her. Simple methods could heal, she discovered.

Martha began to make dietary suggestions to her patients and to advocate preventive health care as a means of staving off future health problems. But these ideas were anathema to most of her patients. They listened politely to her dissertations on diet and the effects of the mind on health, but what they really wanted was a pill or an injection.

In 1980 Martha took the job of director of student health at the New York Fashion Institute of Technology, part of New York State University, and then accepted a fellowship at Mount Sinai School of Medicine's Department of Community and Preventive Medicine. She resumed her post at the Fashion Institute of Technology, incorporating the techniques of preventive medicine, diet, and psychoneuroimmunology.

That year Martha discovered the local macrobiotic community and in the fall of 1983 offered her services as a medical doctor to the local macrobiotics center, either as a teacher or in counseling patients on the diet and life-style. The person she talked to was Neil Stapelman, who, with Shizuko Yamamoto, a longtime shiatsu massage therapist and macrobiotics teacher, ran the Macrobiotic Center of New York. Martha was particularly interested in studying with Michio and Aveline Kushi at the Kushi Institute in Boston. Neil said he would discuss her interest with Michio.

In February 1984 Martha received a telephone call from Lawrence Kushi, who explained that he and his father were designing a small pilot study to follow the blood values of men with AIDS who were practicing the macrobiotic diet in New York. They needed a medical doctor to follow the clinical course of the men and to draw blood from them periodically. Would she be interested in participating in the study?

Martha was thrilled with the idea. She had already begun to deal with the problem of AIDS at the Fashion Institute of Technology and was grateful for the opportunity of participating in a study that might offer some nontoxic approach.

Lawrence had found the doctor he was looking for, but before he hung up he cautioned Martha about what she was getting herself into. "This may cause you some difficulties with your colleagues," he warned.

"That's not a problem," said Martha. "I've been used to following my own drummer for quite some time."

Shortly thereafter she received a telephone call from Michio, who asked to see her in New York. The two arranged to meet in March at a midtown coffee shop.

Now Martha waited for Michio, who finally came hurrying into the coffee shop to join her. Martha ordered tea. Michio ordered black coffee. Michio loved coffee and cigarettes. They were his favorite and most consistent indulgences outside the macrobiotic diet. He made no excuses for either one. He never claimed that cigarettes were good for him or anyone else, and he never hid his enjoyment of them, either. Michio's perspective was consistent with everything else in his life: he never pushed for perfection, only balance. He maintained that every person had front and back, strengths and weaknesses, good and bad qualities, yin and yang. Happiness was attained by achieving balance between one's higher and lower natures. Anyone who sought perfection by repressing all desire usually became possessed by desire—thus achieving the exact opposite of what was sought in the first place. For this reason he never condemned anything or anyone in life. Some said he was merely rationalizing a bad habit, which did harm to his public image, especially as one who promoted health. Michio admitted that it hurt public relations, but he refused to hide his weaknesses or make a great fuss over them. So now he enjoyed his coffee and focused on the task at hand.

He outlined the plan that he and Lawrence and Elinor Levy had designed with the cooperation of the Wipe Out AIDS group. The men would practice the diet as best they could; they would meet regularly at the Macrobiotic Center in Manhattan, where they would receive regular support and information about the macrobiotic program; Martha would provide regular medical advice to the men and draw blood. The blood samples would be shipped via Federal Express to Boston University, where Dr. Levy would analyze the samples and provide the results.

There was no money to do the study. Elinor Levy was donating her time and her laboratory at BU. She was able to do this because she had received a grant to work on AIDS-related research, which she was sharing with the macrobiotics study group. Michio was personally paying for the blood to be shipped overnight from New York to BU. The question was whether Martha could provide medical advice to these men, including the drawing of blood, without pay. Martha told Michio she would donate her time and the use of her office facilities.

All the elements were finally in place. They were ready to begin.

n May 1984 ten men from Wipe Out AIDS volunteered to participate in the study. They would begin to meet weekly at the Macrobiotic Center of New York, located at 611 Broadway in lower Manhattan. All ten had been diagnosed with AIDS and Kaposi's sarcoma. None was expected to survive for long.

The central members of the group—John Angelo, Richard Medrano, Max DiCorcia, and Gary Marks—had already exceeded expectations. (Because Oscar Molini had left for Florida, he did not take part in the study.)

These ten men would form the core of the study group, which would officially grow to as many as twenty. But the original ten were by far the most committed, according to Elinor Levy.

"We added people to the study from time to time," said Dr. Levy. "But most of them were much less committed than the original ten. Some of the people who joined the study later came because they had heard about macrobiotics and the study and were interested in finding out more. But many of them were never committed; they would just stop showing up one day and we'd never hear from them again. The first ten really initiated the macrobiotic program, and they were very committed."

As the program gained wider attention in New York, the support group grew to as many as sixty. Most of these men had been diagnosed with AIDS or came to macrobiotics to give support to a lover who had AIDS. However, the majority of them practiced the diet on their own, or not at all, and records were only kept on twenty men in the study.

One member of the original ten was Steven Jackson, who had been diagnosed with AIDS and KS that previous February. At the time of his diagnosis, Steven was twenty-eight years old. He had grown up in the Midwest but came to New York City in 1978. He found a job as a waiter and an apartment on the Lower East Side of Manhattan.

Steven was raised by abusive, alcoholic parents. His childhood was a series of ugly traumas, brought about mostly by the alcohol-induced insanity of his mother and father. They were physically violent and psychologically abusive. Steven was their target, the outlet for their rage.

As he grew older, Steven developed the looks of a male model—blond, blue-eyed, and handsome. He was also a natural athlete and could run four or five miles almost as if it were a walk around the block. He was an immensely sensitive youth who took joy in living. Despite the abuse he endured from his parents, Steven never stopped loving them, which made the conflicts with them all the more difficult for him to handle.

Steven's life was ruled by a series of profound contradictions. His parents, who when sober claimed to love him, were the most violent and abusive people he had ever encountered. The two most powerful and influential people in his life were the two people most out of control. But the contradictions he had to deal with did not all come from outside himself. He too was ruled by the curse of paradox. On the one hand, he enjoyed being thought of as a minor superman with looks, personality, and athletic stamina—and often felt he could do it all and have it all. But by the time he reached teenage years, he realized that he was sexually attracted to other boys, which made him crazy with self-doubt, self-hatred, and secrecy.

He grew up living a Jekyll and Hyde existence: the perfect

person publicly, the sexual deviant privately. The small mid-western town where he was raised only served to heighten the conflict. The one place that might provide him with the freedom to be himself was New York. But once he got to the city, he lost control of his life.

Steven was possessed by sex. Shortly after arriving in Manhattan, he took up residence with another gay man who became his lover and remained with him through most of the next six years. But such companionship did not stop him—indeed, could not stop him—from rampages of anonymous sex. His most frequent venue was the public restroom, and his appetite was insatiable. No matter how much guilt or remorse he felt after each episode, in a matter of hours—at most, a day—he was prowling the street corners or restrooms again. He was obsessed. He tried repeatedly to stop, but he simply couldn't. He was addicted to the small euphoria he got from such behavior. It seemed to be the only thing that could fill the emptiness that dominated his life.

Ironically, he hated himself while he was engaging in such sex. It was so deeply unpleasant, often repugnant. He was giving himself away to the worst sort of degradation. The part of him that was struggling to survive, to be honored and respected, screamed out against each self-destructive act. Yet the craving for that little gift of euphoria was overpowering.

Steven was consumed with the question of what it would take for him to stop. What was all of this leading to, where was it going, what terrible thing would befall him to restore some sanity to his life? he wondered.

In August of 1982 Steven noticed a strange sore on his leg. It was a lesion of some sort, he knew. Perhaps it was the "gay cancer" he had been hearing about. The thought terrified him and kept him from seeing a doctor until February 14, 1984, when he finally relented, simply because the lesion had been joined by other symptoms—night sweats, swollen lymph glands, and periods of profound weakness. The physician took blood tests and a biopsy of his lesion and within two weeks told him what he already knew: he had AIDS.

He had heard about macrobiotics from some friends who were practicing the diet and life-style. He told his friends of his diagnosis and was promptly encouraged to call Kezia Shulberg for help in starting the diet.

Kezia advised Steven and helped him with cooking classes. In March she recommended he see Michio Kushi for a consultation. Steven arranged an appointment with Michio and went to Boston that month.

Michio examined Steven and gave him the same instructions he had given Oscar Molini and countless others, but he asked another question as well.

"Have you ever thought of coming to Boston to study macrobiotics?" Michio asked him. "You could be a very good teacher."

Steven was greatly flattered. Michio was a man of rare perception, and he obviously saw something in Steven that was out of the ordinary. Steven treasured Michio's suggestion. It was confirmation of a potential he had glimpsed in himself but had never been strong enough to develop. He thanked Michio but said he couldn't leave New York yet. He said he would think it over, however.

"How long will it take for me to get better?" Steven asked.

"If it was me, maybe six months," Michio said.

Steven understood this to mean that Michio had excellent-quality food and cooking available to him so that he could easily maintain the diet, but Steven would have to go through a natural trial-and-error period. He also understood that it was Michio's way of saying that Steven's condition was not so bad.

"You can do it," Michio said.

Steven was both relieved and elated. He thanked Michio again and assured him that he would do his best. They shook hands, and Steven returned to New York.

Now he was part of Elinor Levy's study and determined to overcome his diseases—which, he had decided, stemmed from an obsessive self-hatred.

The first blood drawings for the original ten took place that May at Martha Cottrell's private office in Greenwich Village near

Washington Square. The blood analysis included a complete lymphocyte count, as well as a determination of the ratio between T4 and T8 cells.

T4 cells are the immune system's master coordinator, the cells that direct the attack against an invading pathogen. T8 cells call off the attack. T8 cells are often referred to as suppressor cells, because they turn off the immune system once it has been launched against an invader. In a healthy immune system, T4 cells outnumber T8 cells. Indeed, T8 cells come into action only after the battle has been won, thereby shutting down the immune response so that white cells will remain in balance with other cells in the blood and tissues.

AIDS destroys T4 cells; at the same time, T8 cells multiply, thus suppressing any existing immune response.

Martha Cottrell's initial blood test would serve as a baseline, or standard, against which all future blood tests would be compared to demonstrate an increase or decrease in lymphocyte cells.

Once the group was established and the study under way, Michio and Aveline made monthly trips to New York to meet the men, answer any questions they had about macrobiotics, and encourage them in their regimen. On each trip to New York, the Kushis spent several days giving lectures on everything from diet and health to spiritual growth; Aveline provided cooking classes, while Michio gave private counseling sessions to each of the men. Most of the public presentations were held at the Macrobiotic Center of New York, the Lesbian and Gay Community Center, Public School 41 in Greenwich Village, and Hunter College in Manhattan. Private counseling was done at one of the hotels or at the Macrobiotic Center of New York. Michio saw a continuous stream of men, some with AIDS, some who feared contracting the disease.

The Kushis' commitment to the group, as well as to anyone else who wanted to adopt macrobiotics for any reason, was nothing less than devoted. Anyone who wanted advice or encouragement had only to show up at the support group meeting after a public lecture. There the Kushis would be, very often with Martha Cottrell and Elinor Levy, dispensing information, advice, and inspiration.

There were numerous times, however, when the Kushis could not be present. Then the group turned to the New York macrobiotics leaders, most notably Shizuko Yamamoto, Neil Stapleman, and one of the three senior counselors who came regularly to New York—Bill Spear, Denny Waxman, and Murray Snyder. Stapleman handled the logistics of running the center and making sure counselors were available to the men. Meanwhile Spear, Waxman, Snyder, and Shizuko Yamamoto, a macrobiotic teacher for more than twenty-five years, provided ongoing guidance and support, especially during times of crisis.

"They really kept the whole thing together," said John Angelo. "They gave of themselves. They were there for people consistently. If we hadn't had the center—someplace to go to get advice—there would have been nothing. People would have practiced incorrectly; they would have gotten sick; and the whole idea of what macrobiotics is would have been wrong."

On June 10, 1984, the Kushis held a six-day residential program at the Kushi Institute in Becket, Massachusetts, located in the Berkshire Mountains. It was not designed specifically for men with AIDS and, indeed, was open to anyone with an interest in macrobiotics. Twelve men from the New York support group decided to attend the program; among them were John Angelo, Richard Medrano, Jim Fouratt, Max DiCorcia, and a new member of the support group named Jay Johnson.

Jay had not been diagnosed with AIDS. He had begun attending the Wipe Out AIDS meetings in October 1984, after he met Jim Fouratt at a 12 step program. Fouratt had encouraged him to begin attending the meetings and eventually introduced him to Michio, Elinor Levy, and Martha Cottrell. Since Jay had not been diagnosed with AIDS, he could not take part directly in the study, though he did attend virtually all of the support group meetings and the programs put on by the Kushis.

How Jay had escaped AIDS was a miracle in itself. He was a promiscuous gay man and an IV drug user, with a heavy addiction to heroin and cocaine. He refused to take a blood test because of his fear and his certainty that he was now doing everything possible to maintain his health. He told himself that what he didn't know did not contribute to his paranoia.

The dozen men rode the Peter Pan Busline from New York to Massachusetts. A party atmosphere overtook them as they exchanged repartee on their way into the country. But the shadow of death hovered nearby in the person of one man, Bill Wellington, who at the age of thirty-nine was the sickest among them.

Bill had AIDS, Kaposi's sarcoma, and lymphoma that had caused a tumor on his neck the size of a grapefruit. It was a hideous mass that could not be hidden, especially by the light spring clothing he wore. His pale face and straw-colored hair only accentuated the message of disease. Bill was not a member of the study group, though he did adopt macrobiotics and attended several programs put on by the Macrobiotic Center of New York.

When the group arrived in Becket, Bill was exhausted. The minute he got off the bus, he had to lie down on the sidewalk in the center of town. One member of the group called the Kushi Institute and requested that a car be sent to the bus stop so that Bill could be driven to the institute. Meanwhile local townspeople passed by him as he lay on the ground and cast suspicious glances.

A van arrived and the men were driven along the winding country roads and a long dirt path that led to the Kushi Institute. The grounds were beautiful: six hundred acres of rolling hills covered with tall trees. The view in all directions was utterly breathtaking. The house and the grounds were cupped in the huge hands of the Berkshires, which were old, round, and proud. All around the estate, the mountains seemed to serve as a bulwark against the rest of the world, bathing the place in serenity. The only opening in the forest was to the northeast, where the hills parted in a long, narrow valley that ran as far as the eye could see. The Kushis had purchased the property from the Franciscan priests, who had maintained a dormitory and a rectory house on the grounds. The main house, a grand old Victorian, was now used for cooking classes and staff quarters. The dormitory provided rooms for students and a lecture area.

Once they were settled in, Richard and Robert—both artists with highly developed aesthetic tastes—immediately set about rearranging all the furniture and paintings in the main house. They filled the house with flowers and plants garnered from the surrounding property. Red-and-white rhododendron; bright yellow daisies; white, pink, and red petunias; irises and lilies; wildflowers and greenery. When Aveline walked in, she clasped her hands together and, with a big smile, pronounced it "beautiful."

Meanwhile, Max used rocks and mud to dam up a small river that ran on the grounds, creating a pool for the men to swim in. When the splashing around had finished, the men went back to the house for a hearty dinner.

Bill Wellington didn't join them. He took a separate room and asked for his meals to be brought to him, which they were. He didn't join the group the next day, either, and as the week wore on, his absence became a presence in itself. He was the man not with them, the man they couldn't forget.

The next six days were a cram course in macrobiotic philosophy. The mornings began with an Oriental exercise called Do-In, which is based on the principles of acupuncture. Do-In involves massage and stretching exercises that are meant to move energy more freely in the body along specific pathways that acupuncturists call meridians. Following the Do-In class, Aveline led the group in chanting various Buddhist sutras, or prayers. Later she gave cooking classes and led walks through the forest to forage for wild foods. She directed the men through a world they never dreamed existed, a world of edible plants that grew wild in virtually any moderate climate. She also added her personal thoughts on each plant, how the forces of yin and yang combined to form the plant, providing it with both artistry and utility for human health. As she walked along the forest paths, Aveline found an endless variety of foods that, to the untrained eye, would have been nothing more than uninteresting weeds. As she spoke of each plant, always showing her deep respect for its beauty and natural properties, she revealed its value. Once she came upon some burdock root growing wild near a clump of trees. "Ah, look at this," she said. "Look how strong this plant is, how tough its skin. And yet it can be a sweet and delicious food when cooked with carrots." Then she described the traditional medicinal properties, relating each one to the natural strength and structure of the burdock root. Burdock has long been regarded as a healing herb and a blood cleanser; it is viewed in traditional medicine as a food that strengthens the intestines (known traditionally as the roots of the body), kidneys, and skin. As they went deeper into the woods, the little group came upon a flowing brook that provided watercress—wonderful in miso soup; an open field yielded plantain and dandelion, the latter a bitter herb that traditionally has been used to assist the liver and heart. Other greens were found, each possessed of its own wonders. Finally, some wildflowers were picked to help set the table. At every step along the way, Aveline revealed the magic of the plant kingdom, its beauty and healing properties.

The men spent a lot of their time taking care of one another. The Kushis had taught them to apply various compresses to their Kaposi lesions. They also gave each other massages and brought food to members of the group who wanted to rest. A general concern for one another pervaded the group, a concern that was heightened each time Bill made one of his rare appearances or asked to have his meal delivered.

As the days passed, Bill seemed to need more attention. After appearing briefly at a class or for a walk in the woods, he retreated to his room and requested personal attention from the members of the group or institute staff.

"It's hard to know what a disease does to a person's mind," recalled Jay Johnson. "Up until the time we got to Becket, Bill seemed able to take care of himself, but once there he needed more and more attention. It was as if he had just given up."

As much as people tried to shut Bill's condition out of their minds, they couldn't. More than one member of the group wondered if he weren't some dark metaphor for what each of them would experience.

Richard Medrano, who suffered from a particularly malignant form of Kaposi's sarcoma, behaved in a completely different way. Although the cancer was taking its toll on him, and he would disappear for periods just to rest or attend to his personal needs, he would always rejoin the group later, his attitude upbeat. When asked about his absences, he'd reply, "Oh, I just needed a little extra rest."

In addition, Richard was regularly caring for others in his quiet, understated way, providing compresses, giving massage, getting someone his meals, or offering an uplifting word. Sometimes he would drop in on Bill and tell him of the day's events or bring him some food. People were avoiding Bill as much as they could; his physical appearance, especially the presence of the tumor on his neck, frightened them. More than that, he cast a dark shadow over the atmosphere of hope. Richard didn't seem to be afraid of him, though, nor of anyone else who was in desperate straits. Without making much of it, he often simply disappeared to be with Bill for a while and then returned to the group.

"Richard was very inspirational for everyone," said Jay Johnson. "You knew that he was weak. He had very bad KS [Kaposi's sarcoma]. The lesions covered his entire body, but he was always upbeat, very positive, and very sincere."

John Angelo provided similar support for each member of the group. But unlike Richard, John felt a need to keep others on the right track. It was part of John's nature, and very much his role in the group dynamic, to be more of a pusher and cheerleader than Richard. John was a bit of a den mother; he watched over the others and tried to keep them adhering to the diet. He tried to keep everyone's spirits up. He made jokes and prodded people to be honest about their fears and to have hope. He was also rigorously honest about his own concerns, and his openness prompted a sharing of fears.

One night when John, Richard, Jay, Max, and a few other

men were up late talking about issues of life and death, John made a startling series of revelations.

He had been married for fifteen years before he finally gave up his heterosexual life-style for the gay life of New York. He had had two children, a boy and girl. The boy had just graduated from college, and his daughter was about to be married.

"Two years ago, when I was first diagnosed, I prayed all the time that I would be allowed just two years to see my son get through college and see my daughter through some difficult problems she was having," John said. "And now I've had those two years. And they have been good years, far better than what I had expected when I was diagnosed. My kids are fine, they're on their own. Now I realize that I'll probably live more than two years; maybe I've got another year or two, maybe three, or five or six. Who knows?

"It's very powerful and humbling when your prayer is answered. It makes you really think about your life, about what you are doing. And I'm wondering what I'm going to do with the time I've got left. I look at Bill and I realize how precious time is. Any one of us could have been in his shoes, and we're kind of denying that; but if we stop denying, we might be able to really appreciate what we've been given. Maybe we would know what we're going to do with the time we've got left. Time gets more precious when you know it's limited. I think most of us have faced that. Maybe we can make the most of it.

"I've got a lot of regrets about my life," John continued. "I made a mess of my family. I regret the disco life, all the drugs, alcohol, and meaningless sex. But I'm really grateful that I'm still alive and that my kids still love me."

At that point, John couldn't hold back the tears. Richard got up and embraced him.

After Michio's lecture, the men got together in smaller groups of twos, threes, and fours to discuss the day's events and to sift through the many ideas Michio and Aveline and the other instructors had imparted.

"There was a very positive feeling among us all," said Jay

Johnson. "Everyone was giving a lot of attention to one another, and people had the feeling that they had really discovered something important in macrobiotics. People were hopeful."

In the afternoons and evenings, Michio taught the practice and philosophy of macrobiotics. One such class—on the origin and destiny of humanity—would open up new realms of consciousness for each of the men.

The infinite universe is composed of energy moving in all directions, Michio began. Rivers of energy collide and interact, forming spirals. These spirals produce phenomena, some of which are comprehensible to our senses: galaxies, novas, stars, solar systems, and planets. But everything is composed of spirals, right down to the tiniest particle, the atom, which itself is a spiral of energy and matter.

Spirals are made possible by the forces of yin and yang. First, yang causes the attraction and interaction of two energies. Once joined, yin (expansion) causes the spiral to radiate outward, sending energy to its periphery.

Each thing that comes into existence does so according to the laws of yang and yin, centripetal force causing contraction, centrifugal force causing expansion. The Earth, for example, spins on its axis, creating a centripetal force that we know as gravity. At the same time, its rotation gives rise to a centrifugal force, which throws off energy to create the Earth's environment.

The solar system is a vast spiral, with the planets inhering to the sun by virtue of its yang, or centripetal, power, but remaining at a distance by virtue of the yin force, or solar energy, thrown off by the sun. Energy moves in a spiral pattern. This spiral movement of energy is revealed throughout our own human body. At the top of the head, we have a spiral from the downward-flowing energy emanating from heaven. Energy moves downward along specific pathways and emerges from our hands, causing spirals at our fingertips. Spiral patterns can be seen in sea animals, such as starfish and shellfish; it can be seen in the lines etched in the trunks of trees, in the patterns of flowers, and, most remarkably, in the very genetic composition of human life—the DNA molecule, which is composed of the double helix, or two spirals balancing each other perfectly.

All creation can be viewed as one gigantic spiral, Michio said. This spiral can be seen as having seven levels, or radiants, from the center. At the most peripheral, or most yin, is the absolute world of undifferentiated energy, the infinite source of all things. The next level down toward the center of the spiral is the world of polarization, of yin and yang, space and time, positive and negative. This world makes phenomena possible. Here, yin and yang are interacting as opposites, always seeking balance and peace. The third step toward the center is the world of energy or vibration, including light. Once yin and yang are in existence, energy is possible. Polarity produces opposite pairs, which attract, thus creating movement and energy. The movement of energy causes spirals to form, which in turn produce the fourth world, the world of preatomic particles, the building blocks of matter. These building blocks form the fifth world, the world of elements. Elements give rise to the sixth world, the vegetable kingdoms. The seventh level, the center of the spiral, is the animal kingdom, which culminates in the human race.

The spiral of creation flows from the infinite undifferentiated energy—God, or the Infinite Universe—toward the center of the spiral, the human being. Each step is connected and dependent for its existence upon the step before it. In fact, they are so intimately joined as to be one. There is no separation, no break between God and human. Each place on the spiral gives rise to the next phase of evolution, and each step affects the next form of phenomena.

How, then, can anything happen in the universe that is random? Michio asked. There are no accidents in the universe. There is no mutation, no event that isn't consistent with everything else. Randomness and separation are delusions. All events in the universe are joined; they are meaningful; they are one. You, he said, are one with God.

At the center of the spiral, humanity has no place to go but back toward infinity. The great yangization that resulted in the creation of human life now turns toward its opposite, with an overpowering attraction between humans and the One Creator, the Infinite Universe. The awesome yin became yang—undifferentiated energy becomes matter and human existence; human existence now turns toward the Infinite Source of All.

This is human destiny: to be reunited with the Ultimate Truth or Existence, with the Infinite God.

But in a very real sense, continued Michio, everything that has ever come into existence is still united with the Infinite Universe. There has never been any separation, nor will there ever be.

Life is eternal. There can be no end to life because its source is infinite. You have come into the relative world for a time. Everything in the relative world is composed of yin and yang, therefore whatever has a beginning will have an end. But your home is the infinite world, beyond time and space, beyond matter and energy, beyond beginnings and endings. Each of us will go back to that world. And even now we are still a part of it.

After you have spent a time in the infinite world, you will return to the relative world. The cycle of life is never-ending.

But something remains consistent, even here in the relative world. That is our dream. Our desires are finite. Our time here on earth is finite. But our dream is never-ending. Our dream is what motivated us to come to this world and what directs us in life every day. This is why we say, "Have a great dream." Adapt to the environment so that you can realize your dream.

What is that great dream, and how should we carry it out? What is the Order of the Universe doing? The Order of the Universe is constantly making harmony and balance. We must strive, also, to create One Peaceful World.

At this point Michio paused and asked the men to recite after him a poem or prayer that he had written many years before:

> We all have come from infinity,
> We all live within infinity,
> We all shall return to infinity,

We are all manifestations of one infinity,
We are all sisters and brothers of
   one infinite universe.
Let us love each other,
Let us help each other,
Let us encourage each other,
And let us all together continue to realize
The endless dream of health, love, peace and justice
   on this earth.

The week ended with a small celebration and a great hope.
But fall was coming fast and, after it, winter—even colder and
harder.

CHAPTER

12

That July 1984, Oscar Molini was riding an old train through the mountains of northern Japan on his way to May Li's dojo, well north of Nigata, the only town anywhere near the remote school. Each year May Li left her home in Hong Kong and held a two-month Buddhist training session in northern Japan. Students from all over the world came to study Buddhism with her and endure two months of rigorous, simple living. Oscar wasn't sure why he was going, nor was he sure what the experience would be like. All he knew was that he was searching for something within himself that he couldn't define.

That something had been growing restless since he had begun macrobiotics two years earlier, but it had recently been galvanized by an encounter with Michael Arlington, Oscar's old lover.

Michael was still living in Atlanta. Through the early part of 1984, Oscar had been in touch with him periodically, and the two agreed to spend some time together that winter. Oscar had been lonely in Miami and missed Michael terribly. His love for Michael had never waned despite the distance between them. It had been more than six months since Oscar had seen him, and he now looked forward to being with him once again.

Michael told Oscar that he would stop off in Fort Lauderdale to see some old friends before arriving in Miami; Oscar said that his parents were planning to make a big dinner for him on the night he arrived.

When he finally arrived, Michael said that he didn't want to go directly to Oscar's house but instead wanted to spend some time at a Miami bathhouse, which was more like a gay resort, complete with hotel and swimming pool. Oscar agreed to pick him up for dinner.

When Oscar arrived at the bath, Michael had already consumed a great quantity of cocaine he had obtained in Fort Lauderdale. Now he told Oscar that he was too high to eat; he had no appetite, a common reaction to cocaine. He wanted to skip dinner and remain at the bath.

Oscar was shocked. His parents had gone to great trouble to make dinner for Michael, a gesture Michael obviously thought nothing of. His only concern was having a good time. Oscar was beside himself with anger.

"What is wrong with you?" he asked. "Why do you do these things? You are forever telling me how much you love me, but then you do something like this, which has nothing to do with love. If you said you hated me, I'd understand, but to behave like this and say you love me . . . It makes no sense."

Michael had no excuses, no explanations. He and Oscar had been through this before. Oscar knew what drove Michael: his main priority was self-gratification, which had become his method of self-destruction. Other priorities may have mattered to him, but none so much as his personal pleasure.

Finally Oscar asked Michael to leave Miami when he was through at the baths. They had not spoken since.

Now, as he rode the train through the northern mountains of Japan, the troubling questions of life plagued him: What is this life about if not to have a good time? Why do good times kill? What's wrong with excess? How does one even define excess?

His study of yin and yang, and its implications of a unified universe and a cosmic justice, had been the resource his mind automatically turned to whenever he considered the troubling questions of life. But this study was a demanding taskmaster; it pressed him to apply the ideas to his life—in his diet, his outlook, his approach to other people, indeed, the very way he thought about himself. The more he studied, the more he thought about the essential questions of life, the more he hungered for more information. And for more experience.

May Li's dojo was a large traditional Japanese house, with shoji screens and a rock garden that was brought to life by a small brook that channeled its way through the grounds and under one section of the house. The brook ran under a room used for meditation, which served to attune one's mind to the sound of the flowing brook.

May Li, who had been friends with the Kushis for many years, was herself a practitioner of macrobiotics and provided only the simplest fare of whole grains and vegetables for her students during the two-month program. The day began early with morning meditation, followed by chanting of Buddhist sutras, after which everyone took a one-mile run downhill along a dirt road. A short rest preceded another one-mile run, uphill along the same road. A breakfast of miso soup and grain was then served, followed by the morning chores, which included gardening, laundry, and cleaning the toilets. Everyone then showered in a waterfall near the grounds, dried off, and headed back to the house for a macrobiotic lunch of brown rice, greens, beans, and a sea vegetable. After lunch, people meditated and then listened to May Li lecture on Buddhism.

Buddhism originated 2,500 years ago in India with the first Buddha, Sakyamuni, otherwise known as Gautama or Siddhartha. The religion spread to China and then to Japan, where it was embraced and incorporated into the prevailing religion of the time, known as Shintoism. The intent of Buddhism, like other religions, is to answer life's essential questions: Why do we live? Why do we suffer? How can we escape suffering? How do we achieve happiness? These are the questions that plagued Oscar and the reason he went to Japan to study with May Li.

For two months Oscar sat through many hours of lectures and meditated many more hours on the Buddhist doctrines he studied. One such lecture, which would form a central theme in his philosophical outlook, was the notion that we are one with our environment. In other words, everything in our lives —our relationships, our physical surroundings, our day-to-day fortunes—is but a symptom of our inner nature.

May Li drove home the point that each person's own personal actions have results that one must live with. These are merely the fruit of one's own thinking and daily behavior. We endure the same problems day after day, she said, because our thinking is stuck in habits, conventions, and delusion. We can change jobs, change spouses, change physical locations, but the same problems keep coming up, because we haven't changed the most essential element of all: ourselves. As a result, no matter where we are, we make the same mistakes day after day, giving rise perpetually to a new round of difficulties, sadness, and trouble. The environment merely serves as a mirror for our personal consciousness, or inner nature. It shows us who we are.

There was another essential dimension: the idea of karma and reincarnation. Buddhism holds that there is no death as such, but never-ending life that returns many times to the earth to go through a spiritual evolution that culminates in the ultimate goal: the Buddha nature. Here one sees truth and delusion in perfect clarity and lives in a state of complete happiness and bliss known as nirvana.

Implicit is the idea of cosmic justice: one endures the consequences of one's wrong actions and enjoys the fruits of right actions from previous lifetimes. By experiencing life, one's consciousness evolves and one gradually emerges from the mists of confusion into the perfect clarity of love and understanding that is the consciousness of the Buddha.

Until one reaches the Buddha state, one must endure the consequences of one's delusions by returning lifetime after lifetime. In the state of delusion, one views everything as separate and limited. A deluded person is governed entirely by his ego;

he sees life as a competition over limited resources. He lives selfishly, is willing to fight for what he believes is his, and has little or no compassion for his fellow human. This is how an animal lives, feeling continually threatened, regarding his fellows as thieves in the night. There is no room for love; war is a necessity.

The Buddha sees all things as united. His life is one with all others. His happiness is greater because others are happy. Therefore, he works for the common goodness of all. He seeks to bring others to a state of enlightenment so that they may be happy with him.

All people have a full spectrum of consciousness within them; each person already possesses the Buddha nature, as well as the consciousness just above that of an animal. For most people, the Buddha nature remains dormant and untapped; therefore their actions cannot bring them any lasting happiness. But the spirit is always free, and each person can turn toward his or her own Buddha nature at any given moment to perform a correct, loving, and spiritually freeing act.

How, then, can we blame someone else for our sickness or our personal losses? What political party can save us from our own false thinking? The spirit is always free, and the Buddha nature is always happy. It is up to us to use the Buddha nature to direct our actions. By correct action, we create harmonious causes. This is the way to happiness.

After the lectures, Oscar and the other students performed exercises to incorporate the teachings into their lives. They joined with a partner for three days of serving each other totally, considering only the other's happiness and security. There were exercises in listening, days spent fasting, three days of silence. When Oscar ceased speaking, the sounds of nature came into greater prominence. He was amazed by the cacophony of sounds in the forest—the rush of the wind in the trees, branches falling to the ground, birds in the leaves, bugs in flight, the sounds of his own feet padding against the ground, the beating of his own heart, the sound of his own blood in his veins, the nuances of music in the brook.

* * *

The Buddha nature moves with the infinite flow of energy immanent in all of life, May Li instructed them. It is the nourishing river of life, the core of reality, the thing that governs movement and rest. There are no limits to this energy; it is healing, life-restoring, infinite, and loving. Within this energy one is protected from all disease, all misfortune, all hardship. One is free, light, and pure. One's mind is clear, one's body strong, nothing of harm or impurity can approach it. One can draw on it endlessly and not lessen its totality. It is beyond names. We call it God, Truth, or Tao. But nothing can describe it.

When one is empty of ego, without ulterior motive, one can tap this energy for guidance and restoration. The students were instructed in exercises that would allow them to experience the flowing energy that is ever-present.

They performed t'ai chi, or a Taoist form of martial arts designed to join one's actions with this central rhythm. T'ai chi is a dance, or a harmony of movement, that is performed by transcending one's mind so that one can put oneself in synchroneity with the universal energy of life. T'ai chi, therefore, is a slow, flowing movement which when performed by a master is inexplicably calming, peaceful, and beautiful.

And then there was volleyball, a game May Li liked a lot. At one point in the two-month training, students had been fasting for three days. Oscar was exhausted, irritable, and slightly depressed. May Li announced that it was time for a volleyball game. Oscar moaned; he didn't think he could muster the energy to walk, much less play volleyball. He asked to be excused, but May Li wouldn't hear of it. He explained that he was worn out, but May Li muttered that that was nonsense and made Oscar captain of one of the two teams. She then admonished him to lead his team to victory.

Oscar dragged himself to the net, but as the game progressed he forgot himself. Soon he was yelling and cheering his team on, spiking the ball and diving for low shots. His team won the game, and he marched off the court exuberant. May Li walked up from behind him and said, "I thought you were tired. Think about that."

When the two-month training was near its conclusion, Oscar and the others were performing a Taoist movement exercise similar to t'ai chi. It was a hot August day and the flies were everywhere. One of May Li's assistants went around to each member of the group and swatted the flies off him or her so that each student could concentrate on the feeling of energy flowing. Oscar focused his mind on his inner being and then let go. He started a slow, swirling movement, a dance that was dictated not by his thoughts, but by some inner feeling that had no need of words. As he sank deeper into the exercise he felt great strength imbue his body, as if he were being filled with energy rather than using it up with his movement. He continued to perform the dance, which made him feel light and happy. He was unconscious of himself entirely throughout the exercise, until, near the end, he realized that there were no flies around him. He saw that they had collected around some of the other students, who were being assisted by May Li's helpers, but not one had landed on him or came near.

A great elation welled up within him, and he was overcome with joy. Some rational part of his mind thought, How silly to be so elated over such an insignificant thing. But the flies only triggered a recognition that had been waiting for him to trip over. Now, he was suddenly conscious of what he had been feeling during the exercise: he was at peace. He felt an over-whelming gratitude, almost a nostalgia, for his life. It was good to be alive, and it was good to be Oscar Molini.

As the exercise ended, tears of joy rolled freely down his face.

CHAPTER 13

As fall turned toward winter, and the life began to wane from the sun, the New York City macrobiotic group faced its first trials with macrobiotics, and especially with AIDS.

Bill Wellington was the first man to die. Not much could have been done for him. The tumor in his neck had continued to grow, and it wasn't long before the last strength in his immune system simply gave way.

A young man named Fred was the first official member of the study group to die. He had been weak and very ill from the start and, after making a brief surge at life, weakened further and finally succumbed. Following Fred's death, two men left the study.

By February of 1988, when Elinor Levy would present testimony before the Presidential Commission on the Human Immunodeficiency Virus Epidemic, nine of the twenty men participating would die of AIDS.

Meanwhile the support group kept growing, as more and more men were attracted to the diet, the philosophy, and the encouragement being offered by Wipe Out AIDS.

Michio, Aveline, and three macrobiotics teachers—Bill Spear, Denny Waxman, and Murray Snyder—came regularly to the city to provide guidance and support. Martha Cottrell committed herself body and soul to helping the men cope with the diet, life-style, and difficulties of their disease.

Part of the struggle had to do with sticking to the diet.

"It was hard," said Jay Johnson. "A lot of us had just come off drugs and a lot of sugar and junk foods. Now all of a sudden we were eating this pure diet. The transition wasn't easy."

As one man put it, "I had to go from being completely self-indulgent to being a semiascetic: from Hugh Hefner to St. Francis."

Fortunately for the men, New York has many fine macrobiotic restaurants. In addition, Gene Fedorko and Allan Burns, both prominent members of Wipe Out AIDS, formed a new group called HEAL (Health Education AIDS Liaison), which provides information on a wide variety of alternative therapies for AIDS and other immune-related disorders. HEAL also provided ongoing macrobiotic dinners at Rutgers Church on West 73rd Street. Eventually the group took up residence at the Lesbian and Gay Community Center, where they dispensed information to an ever-growing number of people eager to find new ways of enhancing their body's ability to ward off disease.

Despite the community support that was growing up around macrobiotics and other alternative methods of healing, Martha Cottrell regularly lamented the inadequacy of her resources. With more staff and a greater ability to monitor the men's progress, Dr. Cottrell believed that more lives would have been saved. Without the funds or the staff to provide food and education, each man was left on his own, to struggle against his cravings and limited understanding of the diet and philosophy.

"A lot of the men who came to the support group meetings and began practicing macrobiotics did so haphazardly," said Cottrell. "Some didn't like seaweed, or something else. Or they would stop eating meat or dairy food and start eating whole-wheat bread and say they were practicing macrobiotics, but they really weren't. In fact, they often had little understanding of what they were doing. I was concerned that some of the men who were following the diet haphazardly would run into nutritional deficiencies. Macrobiotics requires a commitment, especially in New York, where the pace of life is so fast. You have to make a real effort, and that requires that you change existing behavior patterns. You have to embrace the new life, and be conscientious about getting good meals. You can't think only about what's convenient, but what is best for you."

Ideally, Martha Cottrell would have liked to have established a halfway house or a boarding situation in which the men could have their meals provided for them. She envisioned the kind of environment where the men could get medical treatment and macrobiotic education. But no such funds were available. Like the Kushis and other macrobiotics teachers, Cottrell was left to provide as much education as she could in her office or at support group meetings.

The substance people craved most was sugar. "In the past, we ate ice cream or candy or some other sweet food anytime we felt like it," said John Angelo. "No one thought anything of it. I used to love hard candy. But now we realized that that wasn't good for us, and it wasn't serving our long-term goal, which was staying alive."

Just as cigarette smokers are more sensitive to the smell and taste of food after they've given cigarettes up, so too did the men recognize the physical effects of every single deviation from the basic diet.

"As you progressed on the macrobiotic diet, you got more sensitive, so that even a little bit of sugar would throw you for a loop," said John Angelo. "You could feel its effects almost instantly."

Michio maintained that the underlying cause of the sugar cravings was the disease called hypoglycemia, or low blood sugar. Hypoglycemia is caused by excessive consumption of simple sugars, found in candy bars, cakes, and other refined products. When one consumes a candy bar, for example, the sugar content of the food is broken down in the mouth and goes immediately into the bloodstream. The elevated sugar levels in the bloodstream cause the pancreas to secrete large amounts of insulin, which makes the sugar available as fuel. At this point one experiences that rush of energy normally associated with eating sugar. However, because the abundance of fuel is instantly available, it is soon burned. Then the blood sugar level drops precipitously, often below fasting levels. In a short while the brain signals that the body needs more sugar, and one craves another candy bar, a glass of Coca-Cola, or some other high-sugar food or drink.

Whole grains provide complex carbohydrates, or long chains of sugar molecules that cannot be taken into the bloodstream until they are acted upon by enzymes in the mouth, stomach, and intestines. Therefore the body can metabolize the sugar in an orderly way, thus providing long-lasting energy that endures through the course of the day. One is no longer on a roller-coaster ride of energy that ranges from frenzied to depressed.

The effect of sugar versus whole grains is very much like the difference between driving a car rapidly as opposed to steady acceleration and consistent driving speed. When one pushes down hard on the gas pedal, one achieves a high speed for a short distance but consumes great quantities of fuel inefficiently. However, when one accelerates at a slow, steady pace and maintains consistent speed, one achieves an optimal gas/mileage ratio.

To help alleviate the cravings, Michio devised some alternate foods and drinks. One drink he concocted was called "the sweet drink," composed of acorn or buttercup squash, carrots, onions, and cabbage, cut up finely and cooked in water until most of the vegetables were broken down into liquid form. He instructed the men to pour the liquid through a strainer and into a cup and then drink the broth, which provided a relatively sweet taste.

"It's a nice little drink," said Angelo, "but it's no banana split."

As for the remaining vegetable matter, Michio told the men that if they craved bread, they could occasionally (once or twice a week) have steamed sourdough bread, on which they could spread the vegetable base left over from the sweet drink. He restricted the intake of flour products because cracked grain is more difficult to digest and loses nutrients shortly after it is milled. Whole grains, on the other hand, are easier on the digestion and retain their nutrient content longer.

But in the final analysis, the strength of discipline was what people needed most. To bolster their resolve, Michio emphasized the importance of maintaining the diet so that their strength improved consistently. Violations of the diet could undermine months of progress.

When he came to New York, Michio met with the men privately. He also held support group meetings in which everyone sat in a circle and each man shared the details of his personal struggle with the diet and/or the disease. Michio, Aveline, and Martha Cottrell then gave specific, personal advice to help with whatever difficulty each man was experiencing.

Michio hammered home the necessity to chew each mouthful of food at least fifty times. "Those of you who have been to Becket for spiritual seminars know that we eat very simply there," he told the group. "We eat small portions of brown rice and we chew each mouthful one hundred and fifty times. At the beginning of the seminar, when everyone first arrives, we put out a big bowl of rice on the table and everyone eats. Pretty soon the whole bowl is finished. But as we go on with the seminar and everyone practices chewing more, each person finds he needs less and less food. Pretty soon, more and more food is left over. When you chew each mouthful fifty to one hundred times, you are satisfied with less food and you don't have the cravings for sweet tastes so much. The reason is that when you chew grain, the sweet taste comes out and you feel satisfied. Also, digestion is much easier."

Michio stressed another aspect of chewing: the importance of saliva. Saliva, he said, is filled with digestive enzymes and is an alkaline liquid. When food is broken down by chewing and mixed with saliva, the flavors of food are enhanced and the food itself is easier to digest. Moreover, the alkalinity of the food strengthens the body against illness.

"Saliva is part of the immune system," he told them. "When you chew, your saliva is alkaline, so the food becomes alkaline.

This alkaline food goes to intestines, making intestinal environment more alkaline. As intestines become more alkaline, unhealthy bacteria and parasites no longer like the environment; they die out or go out of intestines through bowel elimination."

Michio saw the improvement of the intestines and liver as crucial to the overall improvement of health. He maintained that poor elimination caused the retention of toxins within the bowels. Unhealthy bacteria and parasites in the intestines, he said, gave off waste, which proliferated in the bowels and was carried to every cell in the body through the bloodstream. Miso soup, tamari, soy sauce, and other fermented foods provided friendly bacteria to the intestines, causing enhancement of the functioning of digestion and the displacement of unfriendly bacteria.

Michio had observed that many of the men who suffered from AIDS had had bouts of hepatitis. Moreover, heavy drug and alcohol abuse had damaged the liver. One of the important ways to restore healthy liver function, he said, was to eat properly and avoid fat and sugar. Fat and cholesterol clog capillaries in the liver, starving cells of oxygen and nutrients. Excess sugar turns into fatty acids, which are also stored in the liver and hamper liver function. By eliminating these foods, circulation within the liver is improved; stored toxins can be eliminated from the organ with improved blood flow. Cells are replaced, and the health of the liver can be improved.

Once the intestines and liver conditions improve, the immune system has less to deal with and can therefore turn its full attention to the primary disease.

In every support group meeting, Michio stressed the necessity of consuming foods rich in minerals, especially green vegetables and sea vegetables. Refined foods and sugar rob the body of minerals, which weakens the immune system, he told the men.

Finally, "Sing song every day," he kept telling them. In his private counseling sessions with each man, Michio would ask, "Are you singing a happy song every day?"

Inevitably the men would laugh and say, "Yes."

"Good," Michio would reply. "Keep singing."

Michio's ability to inspire the men with hope was almost magical.

"People saw him as a messenger from God, it's that simple," said John Angelo. "There was nobody really willing to help, and here he comes, not just with a very practical and helpful program, but with this grand vision of life."

One man, whose name was Gerard, summed it up. "All of us were very afraid when we came to see Michio, but he gave us hope. He gave us the feeling that we could do something; before that, all we had was fear."

The basic macrobiotic diet itself was also a buttress against fear. It was each man's practical tool, a daily discipline that kept him grounded and focused on his life-style. Macrobiotics provided clear guidelines to follow; it outlined behavior patterns that would increase the likelihood of health. The diet was a practical means of improving the quality of each man's life and the basic vitality he experienced each day. As a result, it was the thing the men clung to for hope.

Moreover, each man also saw macrobiotics as a spiritual discipline. It gave him a sense of purity or worthiness. He was doing the right thing for himself, both physically and spiritually; therefore, there was reason to feel good about who he was.

The love given by Michio, Aveline, and Martha Cottrell was no less important; whether they wanted it or not, the Kushis and Cottrell had become authority figures. For many of the men, they represented surrogate parents who didn't judge but loved them regardless of their pasts. What mattered was what they were doing right now.

Meanwhile, the support of the Wipe Out AIDS group provided ready guidance and an ever-willing ear. The men gave pot lucks, went to cooking classes, and met privately with one another to share their questions, concerns, and fears.

Many lamented that there wasn't more of this kind of support. The conflicting schedules that regulated their busy lives prevented a greater closeness that all the men yearned for. Moreover, the group was growing. In the early days, macrobiotics was one of the very few self-help programs being offered to people with AIDS. Many arrived at the support group meetings or on Jim Fouratt's doorstep at the eleventh hour of their illness. Meeting each man's unique needs was never easy.

Fouratt remembered one young man who had joined the support group that fall. "There was a Dutchman named Pima who lived with a black man for about fifteen years. Pima was a waiter in an expensive restaurant, and his friend was a male nurse. Pima had AIDS and Kaposi's. He was very sick when he came to Wipe Out AIDS. He had been in the hospital and had received chemotherapy, which made him very sick. When he came to the group, he had decided to throw himself into macrobiotics. But right at the beginning he had this incredible outbreak of herpes that was misdiagnosed for weeks after the symptoms were present. He had to go into the hospital again. His friend was very supportive and helpful to him.

"When he got out of the hospital, he was very sick and afraid. His mother came from Holland to be with him, but she didn't provide any real help. She had had a strict Catholic upbringing and went around saying that AIDS was God's punishment upon Pima for being gay. She said this to him all the time. She was very angry and hated his lover, especially because he was black. The longer she stayed with Pima, the more guilt he suffered.

"The problem was, he was so filled with fear that we couldn't do anything for him initially. He was so terrified that he couldn't hear anything we said. He wanted to practice macrobiotics, but no matter how many times we taught him to prepare the food, he'd still mess it up because his fear kept him from processing the instructions.

"Finally, Richard Medrano began to help him. Richard had this honesty and peacefulness about him. He was also very patient. Richard taught Pima how to cook. In the beginning it was tough. Richard would say things like 'You need a pinch of salt to cook the rice' or 'After the pressure cooker comes to pressure, you need to keep it on the stove on a low flame for about forty minutes.' But after Richard said that, Pima would ask, 'Do you have to add salt to the rice?' or 'What do I do after the rice comes to pressure?' He just wasn't hearing. So Richard had him write down everything as the meal was cooked, and then he would go over Pima's notes with him afterward. Finally, Pima caught on; it was a real breakthrough.

"When at last he got a handle on the diet, we could start to work with him on his fear. One of the first things we had to confront was this guilt-producing relationship he had with his mother. In a supportive environment, he began to feel secure enough to deal with their interaction. Soon he wasn't so overwhelmed by his fear, and he could begin to consider cutting his ties to his parent. We helped him face his own responsibility to himself and see what his relationship with his mother was doing to him. Finally, we got him to a point where he felt secure enough to ask her to leave and go back to Holland.

"That was a very empowering act. He felt his own strength and self-acceptance, maybe for the first time in his life. The group helped him experience that power, and he made a choice. His mother didn't like it. She didn't want to be there in the first place; she had her own guilt about her role as a mother in that situation. She was doing everything very judgmentally.

"Later, Pima died, but he didn't die in the chaos of fear. He died very peacefully and with dignity."

According to Elinor Levy and Martha Cottrell, virtually everyone in the study who adopted the macrobiotic diet had some positive physical response. During the course of the research, Elinor Levy circulated a questionnaire among the men to survey their physical responses to the diet. Their reactions were significant.

Before they began the diet, all the men who joined the study reported suffering at least one AIDS-related symptom. Most experienced numerous symptoms, including chronic fatigue, diarrhea, night sweats, chills, and fevers.

However, after several months on the diet there were marked improvements. Of the seventeen men reporting chronic fatigue, fifteen said their energy levels had improved noticeably. All eight men reporting diarrhea said their bowel conditions improved;

of the seven reporting night sweats, six experienced a reduction or cessation of the condition; and five of the six men reporting chills and fever saw the elimination of those symptoms.

All seventeen were able to return to work after leaving because of the debilitating effects of AIDS. Several were working more than forty hours a week. For men who were perilously ill, these were remarkable achievements.

Though no one could say yet what impact the diet had on blood values, especially on lymphocyte count, preliminary evidence suggested that the immune systems of these men were rallying. They were able to fight off colds and temporary infections and throw off previously debilitating symptoms such as fatigue, night sweats, and chills. The general discomfort from their diseases had diminished. The quality of life for all the men had improved. Suddenly there was hope.

John Angelo experienced a complete return of strength to his left arm, which prior to beginning macrobiotics had been growing steadily weaker. Others experienced similar improvements.

But this was a dangerous point, and few in the group realized it.

"A number of the men who started to get better suddenly let down their guard," said Martha Cottrell. "They became lax about their practice; they got a little too confident and started to widen their diets or travel south for vacations, or go back to their more hedonistic life-styles."

Michio cautioned against this very attitude. In the fall, he urged the men not to become loose with their eating habits; he also cautioned against taking vacations to warm climates during the cold months. He felt the change in climate and temperature would be a shock to their systems, and that the temptation to eat foods not indigenous to a temperate climate would cause additional shock to their immune systems.

As fall turned to winter, there was a general feeling of optimism and hope among the men. But then Richard Medrano suddenly took a turn for the worse.

14

Richard Medrano was born to Mexican-American parents on February 16, 1953, in Wilmington, California. His mother died when he was a year and a half, and at the age of six he moved with his family to El Paso, Texas. His father eventually remarried, but Richard was raised through most of his childhood by his oldest sister, Elisa. He showed an early talent for art, excelled at drawing and design in school, and attended El Centro College in Dallas for two years before taking his first job as a showroom design artist in Dallas. Eventually he made his way to Manhattan, became a vice president for sales and design at Karl Mann Associates, and then set off on his own as a free-lance design artist.

His work attracted much praise, and he won a wide variety of awards, including the Roscoe Award, the design industry's Oscar. By the mid-1970s Richard was designing prints, fabrics, and windows for some of the most expensive clients in town, and he had more work than he could handle. In January 1984 Boussac of France, one of the most prestigious fabric houses in the world, asked Richard to design a collection of prints for their fabrics and wall hangings. It was the first time Boussac's had ever initiated a design collection from the United States.

Richard's Achilles' heel was his homosexual promiscuity

and use of drugs. He maintained a high profile in the New York design world—articles and photographs of him appeared regularly in *Interior Design* magazine and other design and fashion publications—and he moved with a glittery crowd.

He was generous and eager to help others whenever he could. When he first met Richard, Max DiCorcia had no profession; he had only recently begun to extricate himself from the dark world of drugs. The two would never have come in contact had it not been for macrobiotics and Wipe Out AIDS. But when Max approached Richard about learning window design, Richard was happy to teach him. In addition, Richard provided Max with work and contacts. He literally opened the doors to a new life.

Richard had been diagnosed with AIDS and Kaposi's sarcoma in the fall of 1982, at the age of twenty-nine. He began macrobiotics shortly after his diagnosis. People within Wipe Out AIDS looked to him as a source of courage and confidence. Everyone had respected him. His willingness to let people make their own choices made him seem freer himself.

There was a pressure on Richard and John Angelo to be perfect people, to have their diets and cravings fully under control, and to be role models of excellence. But Richard refused to succumb to expectations of perfection. He spoke honestly of his cravings for foods and, when asked, about his concerns for his health.

In the early fall of 1984, Richard began to suffer an increase in the KS lesions on his legs. He also developed a lesion on his face, which disturbed him considerably. He didn't want to make a public statement about the fact that he had AIDS, yet he didn't know what to do about the facial lesion. He considered laser surgery to have the lesion removed but wondered if that wouldn't hurt his immune system. He spoke about his concerns at support group meetings and then went to Boston to see Michio. After the two discussed the pros and cons of the surgery, Richard decided to go ahead and have the operation, which successfully removed the lesion. But his approach to the problem served as an example of honesty for others.

Unfortunately Richard's decline had already begun, and nothing was going to stop the AIDS and Kaposi's sarcoma once they gained momentum that fall. (Ironically, Martha Cottrell would discover later that doctors were reporting an increase in Kaposi's lesions and a diminution of immune strength in patients following laser surgery.) The KS lesions began to cover his calves, upper body, and neck. Another appeared on his face. To hide it, Richard grew a beard. His legs and feet began to swell, and he was in more pain that November.

He considered having more surgery but ruled it out because the lesions were now spreading rapidly all over his body, and he believed that if one or two were removed from his face, another would appear right after it.

By Thanksgiving his legs and feet were so swollen and painful that he began to limp noticeably. Within a matter of weeks, he knew he would no longer be able to hide his terrible secret.

He decided to go to El Paso to be with his sister, Elisa, then forty-four, and her four adult children. They were the only family he had. As he told John Angelo, "I just want to go home and put my feet in the water." Probably he was referring to the Rio Grande, which runs south of El Paso at the border between Texas and Mexico.

On December 10, 1984, Richard was delivered in a wheelchair to his sister and her children at the El Paso airport. He refused painkillers but had regular treatments of acupuncture, which did relieve the pain, but only for short periods. Richard refused to eat anything outside the standard macrobiotic diet that Elisa cooked for him.

He spoke to the Kushis and John Angelo regularly by phone. Everyone tried to raise his spirits, but there was nothing anyone could do.

In February he could no longer walk. When the pain became very bad, he asked Elisa to take him to church, where he could submerge himself in prayer. Since contracting AIDS, Richard had become devoutly religious. He had been raised a Roman Catholic and had returned to his roots. He attended Mass, went to confession, and received communion weekly. The Church was his source of strength. As the weeks and months passed, he would increasingly turn his life over to God, as he let go of his hold on earth.

Before Richard came to El Paso, Elisa had considered questions of God, church, or spiritual matters as irrelevant. Now, whenever he asked her to take him to church, she did it only for him. Personally she was indifferent to matters of the spirit, the Church, or the God it claimed to represent.

She was amazed how much church affected him, however. "Every Sunday," Elisa recalled, "he'd receive communion and he came out of church very fulfilled, very spiritually uplifted. He looked forward to church." All of this struck her as remarkable.

Just after Easter Richard took a turn for the worse. The pain was now unbearable. He was taken to a doctor, but there was nothing anyone could do for him except prescribe painkillers, which he refused to take. The doctor did get a full-time visiting nurse to the house to care for him, which was a big relief for Elisa, who needed help desperately.

The KS had distorted his body beyond recognition. In June he could no longer sit in the wheelchair and had to be confined to his bed. On July 12 he was admitted to Thomason General Hospital in El Paso. He was put on an IV and oxygen. But Elisa continued to bring him macrobiotic food, which he ate exclusively.

Fifteen years before, Richard had had a falling-out with his stepmother, Clara; the two had not spoken since. Once he was in the hospital, Elisa asked him if he wanted to see Clara, but Richard was adamantly opposed to the idea. Elisa dropped the suggestion and didn't mention it again.

Richard's ex-lover, a man named Charles, was also calling regularly. Now Richard asked him to come to El Paso to assist Elisa. Charles arrived two days later.

Throughout the next two weeks, Richard experienced a series of seizures. Hospital personnel asked Elisa if she wanted Richard placed on artificial respirators if he went into a coma. Elisa said no and signed the papers preventing him from being kept alive artificially. Nevertheless, Richard rallied after each seizure and managed to pull through. He remained conscious and lucid.

One day, in the middle of July, he asked to see Clara, who came to his bedside immediately. The two were alone for a long while, and when Elisa showed up, Richard and Clara were crying and smiling and holding each other. They were both very happy.

On July 21 Richard called John Angelo to tell him that he loved him. He also wanted to say good-bye.

He called the Kushis, who were in Switzerland giving a seminar. He reached them at their hotel and told them that he was grateful for everything they had done for him. Before he hung up, he told Aveline, "I'm always thinking of you."

Shortly after his telephone calls, Richard had another severe seizure. Elisa and Charles were present in his room when he went into shock. An IV was inserted and he was provided glucose water, which helped him return to consciousness. Once again he was lucid and peaceful.

"He was all bone," said Elisa. "There was nothing left of him. I started to cry, and Charles started to cry, too. Richard looked at him and said, 'Be strong.' "

After a short silence, Richard said, "Why don't we all start praying."

Richard, Charles, and Elisa recited the Lord's Prayer out loud. Elisa wanted to cry but held it back. "If I started to cry, I knew he would ball me out."

After the prayer was concluded, everyone remained silent.

"I saw him staring at the wall," Elisa said. "I watched his face and I saw that he was seeing something. He had a very profound look on his face, and I could tell that he wasn't staring anymore but seeing something that we weren't seeing. He was so peaceful.

"And all of a sudden, he said, 'You know what, I don't feel any more pain.' "

His legs were itchy now; he bent over to scratch them. Soon his fingernails were full of blood from scratching the lesions. He asked Elisa to massage his legs and give him some relief from the itching. Once again he stared at the wall, and once again his face resumed an expression of both peace and recognition. Elisa rubbed his legs and watched his face. When she finished, she moved up the side of his bed to his head and stroked his hair.

"I touched his hair, and I started to cry," she said.

Richard was still preoccupied with whatever he was seeing in front of that wall. Gradually, as if he were turning toward a distraction that was finally getting his attention, he looked up at his sister and then at Charles.

"I'm going to have to tell you something that you don't want to hear," he said in a voice that was surprisingly strong. "I'm going to have to be by God's side."

That night, Richard went into his final seizure and died just after midnight on July 22, 1984.

Later, a nurse asked Elisa if doctors could perform an autopsy on his body for research purposes. Elisa agreed. But a few days later she received a telephone call from a doctor telling her that Richard's body could not be autopsied. It had deteriorated so badly as to be anatomically incomprehensible.

Following Richard's death, Elisa became a committed Catholic, attending Mass and communion every Sunday without fail. She stopped drinking alcohol and smoking. She became part of a group of divorced Catholics who were reconciling to the Church.

"I'm looking for that God that I now know exists, the God Richard saw that last day," Elisa said in 1988. "I want to find Him."

C H A P T E R

15

E ight of the original ten men were still alive, and they were making remarkable progress.

In addition to these men, there were up to fifty more who had adopted macrobiotics and were now being counseled by Martha Cottrell, Michio Kushi, and other macrobiotics counselors. These men also attended support group meetings and macrobiotics lectures.

The men reported general enhancement of appearance, including complexion and clarity of eyes, and attainment of optimal weight. They were sleeping better, had higher energy levels, and were optimistic. For people who had used drugs and sex as an answer to the pain and drudgery of life, these changes were a revelation. Drugs and sex were powerful stimulants with far-ranging aftershocks; macrobiotics was the gentle way, the slow way, to be sure, but it was clearly paying off.

In light of the changes wrought by the diet, the kind of lives they had led in the past seemed violent and bizarre to the men now. Their present way of life opened them to much finer stimuli, gentler vibrations. They became sensitive to their bodies; small changes in diet or behavior could be easily perceived.

"You knew why you had a headache," said Max DiCorcia. "It wasn't something that just happened to you anymore. Headaches were caused by something you had eaten or done the previous day, or hours before, and you knew the cause."

"Before macrobiotics, life was made up primarily of a lot of noise," said John Angelo. "There was so much drugs and sex; it was like chaotic, loud music. After macrobiotics, life seemed to settle down, it became more sane, more relaxed, peaceful. I started to be drawn to more stable relationships. It was like classical music."

The power of the food and its effects on their health gave the men a sense of control that, before their encounter with macrobiotics, would have seemed impossible, especially in light of the severity of their disease.

Jim Fouratt noted that macrobiotics gave the men a daily discipline upon which to ground their lives. The diet and the philosophy served as a guiding life-style that kept them coming back to a place of balance and centeredness. No longer did the heavy hand of morality or the immediate drives of the senses influence their choices; they considered instead the effects each decision would have on their health.

Martha Cottrell was amazed by their progress. No AIDS therapy to date had had a comparable impact on both the quality of life and the enhancement of vitality and strength. The diet's effects on blood values remained to be seen, but so far the results were clearly positive.

With these small but real signs of improvement as incentive, Cottrell began to search the medical literature for scientific corroboration of the macrobiotic hypothesis. Her research revealed a scientific basis for much of what Michio had been saying.

The evidence clearly suggested that AIDS and other immune-related diseases manifested after the immune system had been compromised by a period of insults and debilitation, especially from daily diet. It also gave support to Michio's larger perspective: that appropriate diet could do much to improve the strength of the body's immune response.

Since 1980, an explosion of information had occurred in scientific understanding of the immune system. Cottrell followed the developing medical literature closely; she also studied the existing research for links between nutrition and immune response. The more she studied, the more she realized that the immune system was an extremely sensitive, incredibly complex organ that carried on myriad functions with awesome precision. Its delicacy and internal coordination could be compared to a symphony; its power to destroy an invading pathogen was analogous to the most efficient army ever assembled. But the immune system was vulnerable: it could be weakened and even destroyed.

The first wall of the body's defense system is actually the skin, which protects against the onslaught of innumerable viruses and other poisons that come in contact with us from the environment. Tears, sweat, and saliva are all employed by the body to neutralize and evacuate invading organisms, dust particles, and chemical pollutants.

When a virus breaches these defense systems and enters the body, it can invade a cell and cause it to reproduce the virus many times over. One's own cells become factories for disease. More times than not, however, the immune system destroys the virus before a person even becomes conscious that he or she has been infected. The system also can deal with cancer cells. From time to time, everyone manifests a cell whose DNA, or genetic code, breaks down and causes that cell to replicate out of control. The cancerous cells are usually destroyed by the immune system before they gain a foothold in the body. No matter what the problem—an environmental toxin, a virus, or a cancer cell—the immune system usually has an answer.

This highly efficient defense system operates in several phases: the immune system recognizes the invading enemy; creates a specific and effective response; wages a highly coordinated battle; and eventually calls off the war, thus returning the body to equilibrium.

Once a virus manifests and the first line of defense has been penetrated, the body relies on a group of large white blood cells called macrophages or phagocytes, which lumber through the bloodstream and patrol the system. These scavenger cells gobble up as many invaders as they can and mark the ones they cannot destroy with a sign, or an antigen, that will distinguish the invader as "not self." This is important because the body must recognize self from nonself to keep from destroying healthy tissue.

The presence of the antigen serves to summon other immune cells, the first of which are called helper-Ts, so named because they are trained to react to disease in the thymus gland before they are set free to roam the body.

As part of a general category of immune cells called lymphocytes, helper-T cells (also called T4 cells) actually direct the ensuing attack. Although they do not do battle themselves, helper-Ts act as military commanders, orchestrating the fight against the invader.

Once set into action, the helper-T cells dock on to the virus, which has been partially digested by the macrophages. The helper-Ts signal the macrophages to secrete a chemical called Interleukin 1, or Il-1, which scientists maintain allows the immune cells to "communicate" with one another. Interleukin 1 stimulates fever and deep sleep. Scientists now speculate that fever may actually be an important first step in the body's efforts to destroy an enemy invader. (Whether the body raises its temperature to make itself inhospitable to an invader, as Michio Kushi speculates, is still unknown. In any event, it is now well established that fever is induced by the T4 cell-macrophage interaction in response to an invading organism. Most likely, sleep is induced in an effort to allow the body to dedicate its energies to the task of destroying the enemy.)

T4 cells then secrete another chemical, this one called Interleukin 2, or Il-2, which activates another type of lymphocyte called the killer-T cell. Killer-T cells destroy virally infected cells by attacking their cell membrane. This keeps the virus from replicating.

At the same time, B cells come into action by making specialized antibodies, composed of proteins, to fight the virus. In an extremely complicated set of maneuvers, B cells mutate and shuffle genes to create the individual antibody to destroy the virus. B cells can make more than one million kinds of antibodies. The T-helper cells help select those B cells with the perfect chemical antidote to the invader and then stimulate them to multiply and produce more antibodies.

Macrophages, helper-Ts, killer-Ts, B cells, and antibodies make up the principle thrust of the immune response.

Finally, the battle is won. The invading organism has been destroyed, and a potent antibody has been created to ward off future encounters with the germ. At this point one is said to be immune from future infection. This requires that the cells "remember" the virus and the appropriate chemical response, but like a giant computer that keeps genetic information on hand, the body's immune record is always available and always vigilant against the next encounter with the given flu or chicken pox virus.

Now the immune system must call off the fight, lest it ultimately destroy healthy tissue and, indeed, the body itself. To call off the attack, suppressor, or T8, cells are called out. These literally suppress the immune response by sending out a chemical that tells T and B cells that the fight is over and they are to shut down their activity. This allows the immune system to return to a state of balance, or restful surveillance.

In healthy people there are generally two T4 cells to every one suppressor, or T8. While the ratio of two to one is the general rule, it can go as low as one to one and still maintain health. This ratio of T4 to T8 cells is important to a healthy functioning immune system.

In people with AIDS, the T4 cells lose activity and decline to a point where they are far outnumbered by T8 cells. The ratio drops to well below one to one. Eventually T4 cells are in such a minority that the T8 cell dominates the system completely, thus shutting down all existing immune response. Hence the body is completely vulnerable to any disease that infects it.

In 1983 the French discovered that AIDS was brought about by a virus commonly referred to as HIV, or human immunodeficiency virus. A year later U.S. scientists confirmed the discovery and continued studying the virus, which they discovered was a type of retrovirus. A conventional virus possesses an inner core of DNA that resembles most other cells, shaped in the familiar double helix, or two spirals of genetic information. This double helix makes the cell capable of reproducing itself. A retrovirus such as HIV, however, is composed only of a single strand of RNA, or genetic information. This single strand of genes gives the virus its own unique characteristics but makes it incapable of reproduction.

In order to reproduce, HIV must invade a cell and use a special enzyme called reverse transcriptase to copy its RNA into DNA. At that point it can use the cell's machinery and begin replicating. Some of this viral DNA can insert itself into the host cell's DNA to become a permanent part of the host cell.

Scientists at the U.S. National Institutes of Health discovered that HIV takes up residence primarily in two immune cells, the macrophage and the T4 cell. HIV can remain dormant in these cells, "hiding" for years before it finally "switches on" to its more virulent phase.

Once it becomes active, HIV begins to take over the DNA in these cells and destroys them. Without the macrophage and the T4 cell, the immune system is rendered helpless. T8 cells naturally begin to outnumber the T4 cells. As the macrophage and T4 cells die out, the overall number of white blood cells, or lymphocytes, diminishes with time. T8 cells suppress any remaining immune response and leave the body defenseless against disease. The infected person usually dies from any number of illnesses, including cancer (such as Kaposi's sarcoma) or pneumonia.

On the surface, this process of infection to disease seems fairly axiomatic; that is, if one is infected with HIV, one automatically contracts AIDS. But that is not the case. Indeed, in 1988 there were more than 1.5 million Americans infected with HIV, but the Centers for Disease Control maintained that approximately sixty thousand Americans suffer from AIDS.

Moreover, scientists recognized that there were varying latency periods. One person might get AIDS immediately after exposure to HIV, but another might carry the HIV virus as long as a decade without manifesting AIDS symptoms.

This was a perplexing piece of the puzzle, one of several in the AIDS picture. Martha Cottrell discovered many more such incongruities as she studied the medical literature and worked with people with AIDS and AIDS-related complex (ARC). (ARC mimics some of the symptoms of AIDS; people with ARC often suffer from chronic fatigue, night sweats, and low lymphocyte counts but do not manifest the severe symptoms of full-blown AIDS.)

Ever since HIV was discovered, the prevailing view among scientists has been that the virus is the sole cause of AIDS. But Martha Cottrell's experience with the disease, as well as a growing body of scientific evidence, failed to support this conclusion.

Cottrell and others maintain that HIV is but a single factor in a constellation of co-factors, all of which are necessary for AIDS to manifest. In addition to the presence of HIV, the most important element in encouraging the onset of AIDS is a seriously impaired immune system. Evidence suggests that the virus can be kept under control for a period of time, a period that varies with the individual. This would seem to indicate that the relative strength of the immune system is the determining factor in how rapidly the virus becomes AIDS.

Numerous important studies have led to this conclusion.

Scientists at Johns Hopkins University in Baltimore discovered that a minority of patients—about five in two thousand—test positive for HIV after exposure but are discovered to be seronegative several months later. These people are apparently able to destroy the virus if it invades their bloodstreams.

Other scientists have discovered a protein in the blood that is capable of warding off the AIDS virus after it manifests.

Moreover, research clearly indicates that the onset of AIDS is the terrible fruit of a long process of degeneration.

Dr. Paul Volberding of the University of California at San Francisco (UCSF) found that people carrying HIV show a sharp increase in HIV-infected cells a year before they develop AIDS.

Volberding's research suggests that something changes in the immune system, making it possible for HIV-infected cells to obtain a greater foothold in the system and to spread.

Another study done at UCSF found that as a person becomes sicker with AIDS, the HIV virus becomes more virulent. Dr. Jay Levy discovered that while the HIV virus is dormant, its relative virulence is small, but as the virus begins to spread, or becomes "switched on," it changes into its more powerful and far more lethal stage. Levy studied a group of men infected with HIV and closely monitored the course of their disease. Interestingly, the AIDS virus did not reach its highly virulent state in the one man who did not become ill; in this man, the HIV virus was kept in its weaker, latent stage.

Like a powerful circus tiger that can be kept under control only as long as conditions are right, HIV becomes lethal as soon as its host weakens, at which time—like the tiger—it begins to smell blood.

Dr. Anthony Fauci, director of the National Institute of Allergy and Infectious Diseases, and his colleagues discovered that insults to the body cause a chemical to be secreted from cells that may activate the dormant virus into fullblown AIDS. Fauci reports that chemicals and other infections introduced into the body cause the secretion of a protein called cytokine from immune cells. The repeated secretion of cytokine, said Fauci, seems to serve as a mechanism that activates the HIV virus to its more virulent state. Fauci points out that cytokine is secreted by immune cells after repeated exposure to "noxious insults to the body," such as recreational drugs and infections. Activation of the virus "does not occur rapidly or overnight" but takes place after a period of "insidious conversion" that "gradually whittles away" at the immune system until the AIDS infection overwhelms the body's resistance. In many people, Fauci states, this process takes as long as five years.

Though it is still a controversial point, many researchers have long suspected that HIV alone is not enough to bring on AIDS. Only after the immune system is compromised does HIV produce AIDS.

This has long been Michio Kushi's hypothesis: that a consistent weakening of the immune system through daily eating habits, drug abuse, and promiscuous sex causes a subsequent weakening of the body to the point that any number of dormant viruses overwhelm the immune system; HIV is only one of them.

Michio includes Epstein-Barr syndrome, chronic fatigue syndrome, and the many other recent and mysterious illnesses in this same pattern. Without a general decline in the overall health of the immune system, such diseases could never manifest, he maintains. They would be destroyed before they were able to gain a foothold in the system.

In the United States, AIDS has manifested primarily among homosexual men and IV drug users. Research shows that both groups suffer relatively high incidences of noxious insults.

In one of its early studies, the Centers for Disease Control (CDC) discovered that gay men with AIDS had a history of heavy drug use. In 1982 the CDC reported that of eighty-seven men with AIDS studied, 97 percent said they used poppers (amyl nitrate); 93 percent smoked marijuana; 68 percent used amphetamines; 66 percent used cocaine; 65 percent used LSD; 59 percent used Quaaludes; and 12 percent used heroin. The CDC also found that as a rule the men were multiple drug users, consistently using a variety of "street drugs."

Poppers and other drugs have long been known to depress the immune function and cause anemia, intestinal disorders, and liver damage. Some studies suggest that poppers may be directly associated with the onset of Kaposi's sarcoma. Drug addiction has long been known to depress immune function; heroin, for example, has been found to deplete the number of T cells.

The introduction of sperm into the male body, especially through anal intercourse, has been known to suppress the immune cells. The walls of the intestines are only one-cell thick. Researchers describe the thin intestinal lining, or mucosa, as having the strength of wet tissue paper. The intestinal wall is easily torn, allowing sperm and infection to spread rapidly into the bloodstream. (By contrast, the vagina is lined with a thick protective layer of mucosa cells that protect against the invasion of sperm and other substances directly into the bloodstream.)

Sperm is a concentrated protein containing purines, ammonia, and other chemicals that can be toxic to the blood and tissue. The introduction of sperm into the blood causes rapid deployment of immune cells, which must be directed away from other infections.

The CDC also reported that 80 to 90 percent of the gay population harbors intestinal parasites. Parasites are cited as a potentially important contributing factor in the onset of AIDS among heterosexuals in Africa and the United States. In Belle Glade, Florida, which has the highest per capita incidence of AIDS among heterosexuals, scientists have discovered that up to one-third of the schoolchildren harbor *Giardia*, a parasite common among homosexuals. Interestingly, Belle Glade residents also suffer from malnutrition, poor sanitation, fecal contamination, and a host of infectious diseases. For these reasons Belle Glade resembles a Third World nation and is often referred to as America's "little Africa."

Intestinal parasites have been dealt with by the gay community with the use of antibiotics. But research has shown that antibiotics have a depressant effect on the immune system. In 1982 W. E. Hauser and J. S. Remington reported in the *American Journal of Medicine* that antibiotics depress at least four immune components.

So many factors increase human susceptibility to AIDS, and the risk is increased in men who have been previously infected with a variety of sexually transmitted diseases (including syphilis, herpes, hepatitis B, gonorrhea, and amoebic dysentery) because these diseases are also immunodepressant.

Michio Kushi has maintained that the immune system is directly dependent upon daily nutrition. Dietary factors, such as fat and cholesterol, vitamins, minerals, and fiber content, all play important roles in the relative strength or weakness of the immune system. He declares that by improving the diet and reducing the number and severity of toxic influences on the body, the strength of the immune system can be recovered.

Working with biomedical writer and researcher Mark Mead, Martha Cottrell discovered an enormous amount of information linking diet to immune function. In fact, the findings reveal that proper nutrition is essential to a healthy immune state.

In general, scientists have long recognized that inadequate nourishment causes depressed immunity and vulnerability to a host of pathogens. Malnutrition has been associated with a wide range of illnesses, from scurvy to malaria to blindness. But research has demonstrated a far more specific and powerful relationship between the body's defenses and our daily eating habits.

Saturated fat has been shown to affect macrophages by adversely changing the cell membrane and reducing its sensitivity. Macrophages, or scavenger cells, depend on the sensitivity of their cell membrane to identify and destroy pathogens. Failure to identify a pathogen renders ineffective this first phase of the immune response.

Once inside the system, dietary fats oxidize, or become rancid. These rancid, or peroxidized, fats further break down into substances called free radicals, highly charged molecules that are extremely reactive within the system. Free radicals destroy DNA and cause cell mutations.

In April 1988, Dr. Joe M. McCord, a biochemist at the University of Southern Alabama College of Medicine told *The New York Times* that "the further along we get, the more we are overwhelmed by the number of disease states that involve free radicals." Scientists at the University of Southern Alabama and the University of California at Davis maintain that free radicals are implicated in a growing number of disorders, including cancer, Alzheimer's disease, Parkinson's disease, cataracts, arthritis, and immune problems.

Free radicals are molecules that have become unstable because they have lost an electron. In an effort to regain the lost electron (and regain stability), these molecules take electrons from other nearby atoms. This sets a chain reaction in motion that literally changes the chemical and atomic stability of tissues.

In addition to dietary fat, free radicals are formed by the

intake of radioactive particles, such as plutonium, cobalt 60, and strontium 90. Fat cells are reservoirs for these powerful and potentially lethal substances, which each day are released into the environment from nuclear power plants, medical industry wastes, and nuclear fallout. Fat in the blood and cells also cause chemical pollutants, such as lead and other heavy metals, to adhere in the body. Both chemical pollutants and radioactive elements become part of the system when the fat is broken down and used as fuel, thus releasing them into the bloodstream. Chemical pollutants and radioactive elements destroy DNA in cells throughout the body, including the immune system. Such toxins are foreign to the body and therefore elicit a response from the immune system. These substances cause free radicals to form throughout the body, encouraging a chain reaction of molecular and chemical changes within cells and tissues.

Fat is a proven toxin. Studies have long established that foods rich in fat and cholesterol cause heart disease, diabetes, and cancer. In addition, fat increases the overall toxicity of the system. In the March 1987 issue of the *American Journal of Clinical Nutrition*, scientists reported that the level of fat in the diet directly determined the amount of cytotoxins (substances that injure cells) in the intestines. A high-fat diet, the scientists discovered, raised the level of bile acids and other substances harmful to cells in the intestines, while a low-fat diet decreased the level of cytotoxins within the digestive tract.

Scientists have discovered that foods rich in beta-carotene (such as broccoli, carrots, and squash) and vitamins C and E are "free radical scavengers," or antioxidants. These foods donate electrons to imbalanced atoms, thus restoring stability to molecules and tissues. Foods rich in beta-carotene and vitamins C and E have been shown to prevent free radical formation and stop the chemical changes that otherwise create havoc in human tissues and immune cells.

Beta-carotene has been shown to have powerful protective properties against the onset of cancer, even among cigarette smokers. The National Research Council of the National Academy of Sciences encouraged Americans to increase their intake of foods rich in beta-carotene to reduce their chances of contracting cancer.

Deficiencies of vitamin A have been shown to reduce the size and number of T and B cells. Iron deficiency has been shown to decrease the effectiveness of white blood cells. Minerals such as zinc, selenium, manganese, magnesium, copper, and calcium have all been demonstrated to dramatically affect immune response.

In a study published in the *American Journal of Clinical Nutrition* (March 1987), scientists reported that zinc deficiencies caused atrophy of the thymus gland and reduced antibody response to antigens. Two groups of infants were compared, one that was administered zinc supplements and one that was given a placebo. The scientists found that the zinc-supplemented group had lower rates of infection and higher blood levels of white cells than the group given the placebo.

That the immune system is dependent upon optimal nutrition is well established. Scientists familiar with the evidence have maintained that diet does indeed play a role in the treatment of AIDS and other immune-related diseases.

Writing in *Nutrition Update*, Dr. Brian Leibovitz of the University of California's Department of Food Science stated:

> Two very important areas of research are being neglected: the control of viral expression and the enhancement of immune response by nutritional means. It is my firm belief that these are the two most important areas to be studied with regard to AIDS.
>
> The nutritional treatment and prevention of viruses, as well as the stimulatory effects of various nutrients on immune response, have been studied at length. The results of these studies suggest that nutrients may actually combat all three aspects of AIDS: (1) the viral infection itself, (2) the immunological deficits caused by the virus, and (3) the variety of infections caused by the decline of the immune response (which ultimately leads to death).

There is no doubt that diet directly and profoundly affects the human immune system.

But daily eating habits also affect the way people feel, which also affects immune response. At the Massachusetts Institute of Technology, scientists have found that food changes brain chemistry. Clarity of mind and mood, states of alertness and calm, are all affected by what we eat.

"It is becoming increasingly clear that brain chemistry and function can be influenced by a single meal," said MIT's Dr. John Fernstrom back in 1979. Since that time much research has been done on diet's effect on the brain, all of it demonstrating that food has a powerful influence over what we feel.

Drs. Judith and Richard Wurtman, also of MIT, have carried on the bulk of the research. They have found that carbohydrate foods, such as whole grains, fresh vegetables, and beans, increase brain levels of a chemical neurotransmitter called serotonin. Serotonin causes one to feel more relaxed, clear-headed, and calm. It induces a state of well-being and general optimism. Serotonin also improves sleep and even alleviates symptoms of depression.

Protein foods, on the other hand, give rise to an alertness response. One thinks and reacts more quickly; there is an increase in aggressiveness and a sense of urgency about dealing with the issues at hand.

This information corresponded with the growing sense of well-being reported by the men in the AIDS study. Certainly the increase in energy and other physical signs of improvement were instrumental in elevating hope among the men, but there were also biological changes, even in brain chemistry, that added to a growing sense of calm and confidence.

Macrobiotics, of course, is a philosophical system grounded in a diet. This philosophy provides the basis for changes in outlook and thinking. Macrobiotics attempts to show the benefits implicit in life's difficulties. It offers a view of life that could, if applied, expand the thinking of those who follow its precepts. The macrobiotic view is essentially that life is a never-ending evolutionary path, every step of which is imbued with infinite significance. Nothing happens in life that is arbitrary or unjust. Indeed, all phenomena are united. The macrobiotic philosophy ties the tiny kernels of grain to the giant spirals of galaxies. As such, it provides a larger view of life and a degree of perspective and order. This view holds that human life is an evolving process that takes many forms; that birth and death are alternating states on an infinite path; and that, in the spiritual sense, death is but a gateway, a birth, into another state of being as alive as any other state. Without a spiritual outlook, life seems little more than a mad pursuit of sensory pleasure, a grabbing for all one can get. These ideas promote a new attitude toward life and, more immediately, toward disease.

Healthy attitudes and outlook are fundamental to recovery. The idea that mind and body are one is no longer a philosophical notion, but a well-established physical fact. The mind greatly influences the body's ability to maintain health and overcome disease.

A decade ago those words were thought by many to be either speculation or flight of fancy. But no more. A whole new branch of science has sprung up called psychoneuroimmunology. Its central thesis is that the immune system is inextricably connected to our emotional and psychological states. What we think affects the way our bodies operate. Our capacity to love ourselves and others, our ability to resolve conflicts, overcome difficulties, and accept life's inevitable disappointments—all these play a major role in the effectiveness of the immune response.

It has long been understood that people who have recently lost a loved one are at greater risk of succumbing to disease and death than those who have not undergone such a trauma. Traditionally we term this "dying of a broken heart." In fact, scientists at Mount Sinai Medical Center have found that bereavement has a deadening effect on lymphocytes. These cells fail to respond in the presence of a virus or foreign body. If the bereaved person survives long enough after the death of the loved one— usually about six months—the lymphocytes mysteriously resume their normal behavior and function perfectly. Emotional

stress appears to be the sole cause of the lymphocytes' failure
to function properly.

Stress has been shown to have wide-ranging and potentially
devastating consequences. It creates hormonal imbalances, el-
evates cholesterol level, causes heart and kidney disease, and
ultimately can bring on death. How effectively one deals with
stress can determine both the quality and length of one's life.

When we think of stress, we often think of approaching
deadlines or moments of intense conflict. But stress can be a
chronic problem, especially in cases where a person dislikes his
job or the people around him, suffers long-standing conflicts
with parents or other important relationships, or harbors deep
dislike or hatred for himself. This type of stress can cause a
steady eroding of immune response.

On the other hand, scientists have discovered that the mind
can be a benefactor of the immune system. Positive thoughts
and images can inspire a restoration of immune response. The
mind can be used to reinvigorate immune cells. Cases such as
that of Norman Cousins, who used laughter and a positive attitude to overcome a terminal illness; the work of O. Carl Simonton, an oncologist who has found that positive attitudes
can help patients extend their lives and, indeed, overcome serious illness, including cancer; and the enormous body of evidence confirming that people who maintain long-standing
supportive relationships live longer and enjoy more fruitful lives,
all point to the dramatic influence the mind has over the body.

Many of the men in the macrobiotic support group were
using a wide variety of positive imaging routines. Most involved
images of being in a peaceful natural setting, alone or with a
loved one. The use of meditation devices varied widely among
the men, but virtually every one of them used some form as a
means of bringing calm and centeredness to the mind and emotions.

Among the most popular meditation and positive imaging
routines were those of Louise Hay, author of the books *Heal
Your Body* and *You Can Heal Yourself*. Her tape "A Positive Approach to AIDS" has been especially helpful to those with AIDS

or at risk of contracting AIDS. Hay's work centers on personal responsibility for the circumstances in one's life—including sickness, misfortune, good fortune, and health. She maintains that all disease is the result of unreconciled emotions, especially resentment, anger, and guilt. Her imaging routines are designed to release these and other negative emotions. To love oneself, says Hay, is the central issue for all people, but especially for the sick, who have brought on their particular illness as a result of their long-standing emotional ill health. Louise Hay is especially appealing because her philosophy and guided imagery routines have a spiritual and loving focus. Many of her affirmations and guided imagery exercises invoke the deity or universal force.

"The Universal Power never judges or criticizes us," is the beginning sentence of one of Hay's positive affirmations in *You Can Heal Yourself*. "It only accepts us at our own value. Then it reflects our beliefs in our lives. If I want to believe that life is lonely and that nobody loves me, then that is what I will find in my world.

"However, if I am willing to release that belief and to affirm for myself that 'Love is everywhere, and I am loving and lovable,' and to hold on to that new affirmation and to repeat it often, then it will become true for me. Now loving people will come into my life, the people already in my life will become more loving to me, and I will find myself easily expressing love to others."

Louise Hay knows firsthand the trauma of disease and personal conflict. She overcame cancer herself, as well as a childhood of physical, emotional, and sexual abuse, by using the methods she describes in her books.

The more Martha Cottrell read and experienced with the men she tried to help, the more frustrated she felt with the medical profession's current approach to AIDS.

"All the emphasis today is on finding a drug to cure this illness or a vaccine to prevent it," she said. "But we have no cure and there is no vaccine yet, and there are people dying.

AIDS must be addressed in a multidisciplinary way. It's the only thing we really have. The data are all there. Diet can be effective in helping restore the immune system. The mind is a powerful tool in the restoration of health. We doctors have to work with all the tools available if we are going to do some good for people who are sick. We cannot harbor silly prejudices in the face of life-and-death questions. There are times when medical intervention is absolutely necessary. Macrobiotics is a slow way, a gentle way, of reestablishing balance, but sometimes we don't have a lot of time; a person is too far gone for macrobiotics to help him, so we must rely on medical intervention to do some good. But there are many people out there who can benefit by this approach, and we should be offering it."

Cottrell constantly lamented her lack of sufficient funds to provide such multidisciplinary tools to the men who came to her for help. She wanted to bring in people who were skilled at positive imaging routines; she wanted to have facilities available to house the men and ensure that proper cooking and food were supplied. She wanted to offer the psychological and spiritual counseling that so many of them needed in order to deal with their long-standing conflicts. In the end, she was left with the reality of her limited resources and those of her macrobiotic friends. "We could only do so much, no matter how much more we wanted to do," she said. The rest was left to fate.

In the spring of 1985, the eight men remaining from the original ten were making clear strides toward greater health. Most of them had been alive for more than two years already and showed no sign of decline. Indeed, from outward appearance, they were healthy and active young men. Most guarded their illness with understandable secrecy, and few of their associates knew they were ill.

One of the changes that assisted their secrecy was the disappearance of some of their Kaposi's lesions. Michio had said that this would happen and that new lesions would emerge from time to time, only to slowly resorb as well. He maintained that KS was a manifestation of the body's attempts to eliminate poisons long stored up within the system, and that the lesions were largely a drug discharge; once the toxins had been entirely thrown off by the body, all the KS lesions would heal and vanish. The men were now watching his words become reality.

In June Elinor Levy took another round of blood tests to be compared with the initial baseline tests taken one year before, in May 1984. These would show the progress the men had made, or failed to make, while practicing macrobiotics.

There was a general feeling of hope and expectation among the men. They had not replicated the typical AIDS patient's course. On the contrary, most had experienced a remarkable improvement of health and now looked forward to hearing Elinor Levy's report.

16

I n June 1985, Elinor Levy announced the results of the blood values to date. Seven of the eight men with Kaposi's sarcoma still continuing in the study had experienced a remarkable improvement in lymphocyte number.

Lymphocytes (the group of white blood cells that include macrophage, T4, and T8 cells) range in healthy adults from 1500 to 3500 per cubic centimeter of blood. A rapid and severe decline in lymphocyte number normally accompanies a diagnosis of AIDS, and that decline generally continues as the disease progresses.

Max DiCorcia was diagnosed with AIDS and KS in September 1983; he met Michio Kushi two months later and adopted the macrobiotic diet. His lymphocyte number went from a baseline of 1368 in May 1984 to 1800 in June 1985. In the course of one year, his condition improved markedly.

Gary Marks was diagnosed with AIDS and KS in September 1983, attended the same Kushi lecture as Max at the Lesbian and Gay Community Center, and began the diet immediately after. At that time his baseline lymphocyte count was 1575 cc. In June of 1985, it had risen to 2900.

Louis Bonadio was diagnosed with AIDS in September 1984,

saw Michio a month later, and immediately joined the study. His baseline then was 1400; in June 1985 it was 1500.

John Angelo was diagnosed with Kaposi's sarcoma in May 1982. Sloan Kettering sent his original diagnosis and blood records to Elinor Levy and Martha Cottrell; at diagnosis, his lymphocyte count was 1817 cc, which Levy used as his baseline. John began the macrobiotic diet a year after his diagnosis, in May 1983. In June 1985 his lymphocyte count was 2560 cc.

Gary Metz was diagnosed with AIDS and KS in January 1985. He immediately began the macrobiotic diet and joined the study group. His baseline test, done that January, was 1677 lymphocytes per cubic centimeter of blood. No June figure was taken, but in September 1985—some nine months after he began macrobiotics—his count was 2160.

(Steven Jackson left the study shortly after the baseline blood work was done and moved to California. He remained faithful to his macrobiotic diet, however, and he continued to be followed by Elinor Levy and Martha Cottrell. Jackson's initial blood test showed a lymphocyte count of 1530. Further blood work done on a visit to New York in March 1986 revealed a lymphocyte count of 1575. He continued his healthful regimen and remained in good health at the time this book was written in the fall of 1988. He was still considered a part of the study group.)

Of the two remaining members of the group, one man remained unchanged and the other showed an improvement in lymphocyte count. Seven of the eight men saw their lymphocyte count return to normal.

Remarkably, these seven men showed a stabilization of T4 cells. Since HIV kills T4 and other lymphocyte cells, AIDS patients typically experience a sharp decline in T4 cells.

In June, Levy, Beldekas, Cottrell, and Lawrence Kushi reported their initial findings in the form of a letter to the British medical journal *Lancet*. The letter was subsequently published in the July 27, 1985, issue. In it, the scientists ask whether it is ethical to offer placebo, or nontherapeutic, medication to AIDS patients. The question is relevant to the Boston University study because macrobiotics is considered by most physicians to be without therapeutic value. These physicians, however, do hold out a slim hope that current therapies might have some impact on the course of AIDS. The letter states:

At the International AIDS Conference in Atlanta last April someone asked if it would be ethical to include a control or placebo group in drug trials in Kaposi sarcoma (KS). The implication was that lack of treatment would reduce survival. This does not seem to be so. Since May 1984, we have been studying immune function in a group which includes ten men with KS who have chosen not to enter conventional treatment protocols. Eight are still alive an average of 21.5 months after diagnosis (range 13—37 months). One person died 11 and another 20 months after diagnosis....

These men seem to be surviving at least as well as patients who have been treated.... Their choice to forgo conventional medical therapy may indicate a strong, independent psychological makeup which could enhance survival. They are all following a vegetarian (macrobiotic) diet and have a strong social support system.... Survival in these men who have received little or no medical treatment appears to compare very favourably with that of KS patients in general....

The letter was signed by Levy, Beldekas, Cottrell, Kushi, Paul H. Black, and Robert Lerman, the last two associated with Boston University School of Medicine.

The men continued to show steady progress over the next six months. In January 1986 Elinor Levy sent Michio a letter and a report detailing the progress to date.

The results of our ongoing study of men with AIDS who are macrobiotic are encouraging.... We have been studying the men sequentially since May 1984 to follow certain immune parameters. At present the data suggest a

stabilization of the % T4 positive cells and lymphocyte
number in about 50 percent of the group. The general
pattern in people with KS is a steady decline in both % T4
and total lymphocyte number. This is thought to be a
significant indicator of morbidity. Therefore the ability to
stabilize these parameters, in so large a proportion of our
study group, is a hopeful sign.

The letter was signed by both Elinor Levy and John Beldekas.

In a detailed report given at the Second International Conference on AIDS, Levy and Beldekas concluded as follows:

1. Lymphocyte number increases over the first two years from
   diagnosis with Kaposi's sarcoma in men who are following
   a macrobiotic diet. A linear regression analysis model predicts that lymphocyte number becomes normal within this
   two-year period.
2. During this time period the percentage of T4 cells does
   not change. The percentage of T8 cells possibly decreases.
3. These results compare favorably with those from any of
   the medical treatments reported.
4. There are several possible explanations for these positive
   findings, including:
   a) The macrobiotic diet and/or life-style is of benefit to
   men with Kaposi's sarcoma.
   b) The decision to become and remain macrobiotic selects
   for men with a better prognosis.

The reaction to these blood tests from the men was one of
muted elation. There was a sense that they could do it—that
they could beat the unbeatable disease. But it was an ongoing
struggle that would not end. There is still no cure for AIDS, but
each man who had come this far believed that his macrobiotic
practice was a defense against death. And more: macrobiotics
had changed the quality of each man's life dramatically.

In the summer of 1988 Gary Marks was still alive, nearly five years after diagnosis; he was still healthy and still working at least forty hours a week at his own business. He summarized the changes he had undergone during those years.

"My whole life has been changed by macrobiotics," he said. "I'm light now; the burden of AIDS is gone. But it's not like I'm cured, either. I look at my disease as if I have a chronic condition; I tell myself I have something like diabetes. There's no cure, but I can live and live well if I'm careful. I have to eat well; I have to take care of myself; and I have to love myself. I have to choose to be positive. For the first time in my life, my brain isn't between my legs, it's in my head. As long as it's there, I have the power to make wise choices. I used to have very low self-esteem. That causes you to do things that are destructive because you think that's all you can get. You don't believe anyone will love you, so you don't seek love. But when you love yourself, you honor yourself; you attract supportive relationships and you choose to keep certain harmful things out of your life. I can't eat certain foods; I can't do certain things. But I'm alive, and you know something, I'm happier now than I've ever been."

In June 1987 Elinor Levy presented her findings at the Third International Conference on Acquired Immunodeficiency Syndrome (AIDS) in Washington, D.C. Her official abstract, which she presented at the conference, read as follows:

Twenty men who have chosen a holistic approach to their diagnosis of Kaposi's sarcoma have been studied sequentially. They are all following a macrobiotic regimen. The median survival for the 8 men who have died is 19 months (range 5–46 months). None of the surviving members of the cohort have required hospitalization. One has required local radiation. Four are alive 3 or more years after diagnosis. Contrary to what might be expected, the number of lymphocytes in the group has increased with time over the first 3 years after diagnosis.... The number of T4 cells increased over the first 2 years after diagnosis.... The percentage of T8 cells was unchanged.... A subset of approximately ⅓ of these patients have filled out the

McNair's Profile of Moods Survey (POMS). Preliminary data suggests these men are generally less depressed ... less anxious ... and feel more energetic ... than has been reported for other cohorts of men with AIDS. The psychological profile associated with this group is hypothesized to have a beneficial effect on the clinical course of their disease.

On February 20, 1988, Elinor Levy presented the same findings as testimony for the Presidential Commission on the Human Immunodeficiency Virus Epidemic. She provided a statement and answered questions from a panel of scientists. In her prepared statement, she stated as follows:

> I will concentrate my remarks on nutrition as a possible co-factor in HIV-related disease. In general, malnutrition is associated with significantly impaired immune response. The immune response is also sensitive to deficiencies and excesses of single nutritional elements, and to the quantity and quality of fat intake. Nutrition can be shown to affect susceptibility to a variety of infectious agents and is implicated in the development of cancer. I have been involved in a pilot study of men with AIDS-related diseases who have chosen to follow a macrobiotic regimen. This includes a vegetarian diet, a healthy life-style, and a sense of hope and control. The large majority report an improved [sic] in AIDS-related symptoms. Additionally, those in the group with KS also show an increase in their number of lymphocytes during the first three years after diagnosis, and six of nineteen men are alive greater than three years after diagnosis with KS....
>
> I would recommend that the NIH [National Institutes of Health] foster more of an interest in nutritional and other co-factors through the organization of small workshops to bring together the multidisciplinary talents needed to work out design and methodological issues, and by encouraging research.... I would recommend that nutritional

components be added onto ongoing "natural history" studies, and/or that new studies focusing on psychological and nutritional co-factors be encouraged, including those with an intervention design. . . .

At this time I cannot give an estimated cost for implementing these recommendations but suggest it would be a modest investment compared to what could be saved in health care and social service costs if onset of debilitating symptoms can be delayed or prevented. Although the state of our knowledge about the factors predisposing to the progression of HIV infection is not extensive, it is extremely likely that co-factors play an important role. There is an urgent need for research in these areas, so that accurate information can be used as a basis for more effective treatment strategies and educating persons at risk.

CHAPTER

17

In September 1986 Oscar Molini moved back to New York City and found an apartment on the Upper East Side of Manhattan. Shortly after returning, he was hired by an architectural firm to handle interior designs. That year he turned thirty-nine years old, and life had settled into a more comfortable and mature pattern.

Despite their many disagreements, Oscar's love for Michael never waned. After the incident at the Miami baths in the summer of 1984, Oscar had decided to stay in touch with Michael but remain at a distance. He couldn't expect any sort of stable relationship from him. Michael was without stability himself—how could he bring it to a relationship? Then, after Michael moved to Seattle in 1985 and took an apartment with another gay man, Oscar decided to let him go entirely.

But two years later he still had a lasting love for Michael. One night in September of 1987, he and Cheryl were having one of their late night talks when Oscar confessed that he still loved Michael dearly and wished that he was in touch with him.

"Then call him," said Cheryl.

"Do you really think I should?" Oscar said.

"Oscar, of course I think you should. Call him now."

Oscar found Michael's telephone number with the help of

Seattle directory assistance. He wrote the number down and stared at it for several anxious moments. How would Michael react to him? They hadn't talked in so long.

Too nervous to call, Oscar decided instead to call Cheryl back; when she picked up the receiver, he heard her baby crying in the background. "Hi, it's me again," he said. "Do you really think I should call?"

"Oscar, don't bother me, I'm busy with the kids," Cheryl said.

Oscar apologized and hung up. Now he gathered his courage and dialed the number. Recognizing Michael's voice instantly on the other end, Oscar stumbled through the greeting.

"I thought you were dead," said Michael. He explained that for the previous year, he had believed Oscar had finally succumbed to AIDS. But he didn't know for certain and had recently begun to make inquiries about Oscar's fate. Michael confessed that his feelings for Oscar had endured, too. He told Oscar that only a few days before his call, he had discovered through a mutual friend that Oscar was fine. That day, he'd called Oscar but after hearing him say hello had hung up.

Oscar was glad now that he had called. Finally he asked Michael how he was.

Not good, Michael replied. He had been in the hospital three times with AIDS and pneumocystis. His health was failing rapidly, and he was afraid. He had tried to return to macrobiotics, but he simply didn't have the willpower. He knew only one way to live.

Michael told Oscar about a big AIDS walkathon taking place in Seattle that month to raise money for research. Michael wanted to participate in it but was afraid his health would prevent him from taking the six-mile walk. He was scheduled to go back into the hospital that week.

The conversation ended with each of them promising to see the other when possible.

Michael went into the hospital that week and was placed on IV. He was weak, but on the day of the walk he left the hospital in a wheelchair equipped with an IV pole and completed the entire distance.

In October Michael went to Washington, D.C., for a walk-athon and rally for AIDS research. At the rally, he made a moving speech to the enormous throng, explaining that he was dying of AIDS and that a cure would not likely be found in time to save his life.

He was terribly weak now and had a temperature of 103 degrees F, but he had found a mission and it gave him courage and strength.

From Washington he went to New York and stayed with Oscar. Oscar was happy to see him, but it was heart-wrenching, too, because Michael was dying.

Despite his failing health, Michael wanted to see the Broadway show *Starlight Express*. Oscar surveyed every ticket outlet he could think of and managed to get orchestra seats for the sold-out show. Michael loved it.

The following night, the two sat in Oscar's living room, talking. At one point they fell silent. At last Michael spoke. "You know what, Oscar . . ." He paused, searching for the right words.

"You don't have to say anything, Michael," Oscar said, reading his mind. "I'm so happy you're here."

"I've always cared," Michael said. "It's just that I was always doing the wrong things. I was always making mistakes."

"You don't have to say anything," Oscar repeated. "I understand. You're different now, I can see that."

The next day, Michael left for Seattle and was immediately readmitted to the hospital.

During the Thanksgiving weekend, Oscar flew out to be with him in the hospital. Michael was near death, slipping in and out of consciousness. When he was lucid, he would flash a radiant smile at Oscar. Oscar was so moved by that smile. It transcended the pain and the trouble they had gone through together. It even transcended the suffering Michael was now experiencing. Oscar had never felt so much love for another human being.

Michael's room was filled with flowers sent to him by friends. At one point he came out of his coma and said, "Oh, isn't it beautiful."

"Yes," Oscar said, trying to be cheery. "The flowers are great."

Michael shook his head. "Oh, no, Oscar. What I'm seeing is not here."

Oscar returned to New York after the holiday weekend, and on December 8, 1987, Michael died.

"I did not know I could feel so much," Oscar said later. "I did not know I could love and hurt so much."

The depth of his feelings for Michael changed Oscar forever. He had known love. It was the most powerful experience he had ever had, and nothing else compared with it.

"When you love someone, they become a part of you in a deep and lasting way, and even when you are apart they are with you, in your feelings and in your memory," he said.

Those memories weighed heavily upon Oscar, however. For weeks and months after Michael's death, he couldn't shake the feeling of loss. "You feel a little bit crippled," he said. "The part of your life that you gave in the form of love is gone."

As 1988 dawned, Oscar became increasingly depressed. He lost his appetite. Food stopped appealing to him. His adherence to the macrobiotic diet slowly diminished.

"I was so devastated by Michael's death that I began to feel tired," Oscar recalled. "I stopped keeping an upbeat attitude. I couldn't keep up the fight. I just plummeted to the bottom. Once that happened to me, I stopped doing the things I should. I didn't feel like cooking anymore, so the quality of my food began to decline. Pretty soon, it didn't taste good to me, so I started to eat outside the diet. And then the whole thing snowballed because I just didn't feel like doing what was good for me anymore."

Michael's passing brought Oscar closer to the whole issue of death.

"When you lose someone you love, you feel close yourself to the next step, especially if you are in the same boat," he said. "It's a struggle against this disease. You have to keep your spirits up and maintain the good habits that you know are keeping you well. But you can get knocked down, and it's like you lost the game suddenly. Every negative thing gets to be five times bigger, and you feel like you're just too tired to keep up the fight."

By the spring of 1988, Oscar's vigilance had completely subsided. He had gained weight; he had stopped caring about what he was eating. The loss of Michael was with him always, like a noxious cloud, poisoning him a little more each day.

That spring he developed a new lesion on his foot, and it began to grow. By early summer his legs began to swell—the first signs of phlebitis. These symptoms worried him. He knew he had to climb out of his depression, but how?

He started to give presentations at the Macrobiotic Center of New York on his experience with AIDS and macrobiotics. At the same time, he took a job delivering food to people with AIDS who were bedridden and could not leave their homes. He worked for a small private group called God's Love, We Deliver, which obtained surplus food from New York restaurants and delivered it to the sick. Oscar always requested that the best quality be provided by the restaurants and encouraged others to come to the HEAL dinners, which each week provided macrobiotic food. In his way he was reaching out, looking desperately for a purpose, a reason to go on living.

In May of 1988 Oscar traveled to Japan with the Kushis and Martha Cottrell to talk to Japanese audiences on the growing problem of AIDS in the United States and what could be done to protect future generations.

Meanwhile, his health continued to decline. When he returned to the United States, the lesion on his foot grew larger and more painful. That summer the phlebitis in his legs worsened. Soon he couldn't walk and could no longer go to work each day. He began to feel weak.

"I couldn't coast along anymore, telling myself that I could start cleaning up my habits tomorrow," he said. Any more waiting and there would be no more tomorrows.

The resurgence of his illness shocked him from his stagnation and depression. Terrified, he went to Boston to talk privately with Michio. He confided that he had let his diet and his positive attitude slip away, and that now his health was in serious jeopardy. Michio was concerned as well. He gave Oscar a strict set of dietary recommendations and urged him to redouble his efforts. But such urgings were unnecessary now. Fear had kicked Oscar's will back into gear. He wanted to live, and he would do anything necessary to go on doing just that.

Now he resumed his quality cooking and pristine diet. In addition he began taking homeopathic remedies and herbs, including eluthero, echanasia, and red clover, all of which are traditional herbs used to stimulate immune response.

Miraculously, the regimen began to work. By the fall of 1988, the swelling in his legs was gone. The lesion and swelling on his foot had begun to diminish as well, and he could resume walking. His energy returned; he felt stronger. He began to take on some part-time design work and was planning a new future for himself. Once again, Oscar was making a comeback.

The process of getting sick again and then starting the long haul back has taught him a great deal, he says. "When I got depressed, I went off the diet and my mind got cluttered up with all sorts of garbage—dark thoughts and confusion. Macrobiotics gives you clarity of mind. If you eat a very clean diet, you can think clearly, and it's easier to make the right decisions about your health. Once I got back on the diet, it was easier to do the right thing again. But when you eat junk and drink coffee, it starts disturbing your sleep; it weakens your energy levels; you feel sluggish, and your energy levels go up and down, and pretty soon you're on a roller coaster. I experience this every time I go off the diet."

In October 1988 Oscar said: "I know I'm on the right track again because I can see it and feel it physically. I'm on my way back."

CHAPTER 18

The year 1988 saw Michio and Aveline Kushi step up their educational activities linking diet to the prevention and treatment of AIDS. They began the year by spreading the word in the places they believed needed it most.

In February Michio, Aveline, and an entourage that included Elinor Levy, Martha Cottrell, and a group of macrobiotics teachers went to Brazzaville, the Republic of Congo, in Africa, to instruct people there in the importance of diet in the prevention and treatment of AIDS. Henri Lucy, a leading figure in the macrobiotic community of France, worked with the Health Ministry of the Congolese government and a medical doctor from the World Health Organization to organize the lectures, which attracted two hundred medical doctors and scientists from all over Africa.

What Michio and his small contingent found there was the horrible scourge of AIDS on a grand scale. AIDS has gone completely out of control in Africa. No one knows the number of people infected or killed by the disease. African governments have repressed that information. In 1987 the official number of cases of AIDS in Africa was 2,627. However, blood tests in Lusaka, the capital of Zambia, show that 18 percent of blood donors are infected with HIV. In Nairobi, Kenya, 67 percent of prostitutes tested have been HIV-positive. In Kinshasa, Zaire, which has a population of four million, blood samples of thousands of residents show that 6 to 7 percent of the general population have been infected. A recent German study forecasts that at the current rate of infection, AIDS will infect 75 percent of Africans within five years.

African health officials willing to talk about the plague point out that the existing health care systems are already stressed beyond their capacity to deliver adequate treatment for the sick and dying. Experts state that rampant promiscuity, genital sores, intestinal parasites, poor sanitation, poverty, and widespread ignorance are among the many reasons cited for the vicious spread of this disease.

Michio and Aveline went into the local villages and talked to the people about their diets and the diets of their ancestors. They toured the countryside and local farms, examining the current diet and asking about the food that was traditionally eaten by residents of the Congo. At one point Michio went to the local rivers and examined the vegetation growing in the streams. He recommended that the people begin eating these vegetables, which he said were rich in important vitamins and minerals.

Immediately several of the natives recalled that their parents and grandparents had foraged the rivers and eaten these foods generations before. But that practice, like so many others, had disappeared with the modern ways of eating and living.

Meanwhile, macrobiotic teachers Evelyne Harboun, Masao Miyaji, and Dr. Fredric Bodin all provided classes for the local people.

At the subsequent macrobiotic conference, the audience was made up of a rainbow of peoples from all nations. Michio laid out in great detail the macrobiotic approach to health and illness, specifically AIDS. He offered his recommendations on what the diet in Africa should be: a replica of the traditional diet of the Congo, made up largely of millet, cassava, vegetables, beans, river weeds, fruit, and small amounts of animal foods. In addition, he urged the people to return to their traditional ways of processing foods, raising their children (including breast-feeding), and maintaining strong nuclear families.

"We must begin again to eat the food our grandparents ate," Michio told them. "We must nurse our babies, eat unprocessed grains, vegetables, beans, and fruit that are indigenous to our regions. We must retain strong family ties and traditional values. Then we will begin to restore our health; we will have the native strength our grandparents enjoyed."

On the final day of the conference, a resolution was adopted by the conference doctors to spread macrobiotics throughout their native lands as part of a public education campaign to prevent and treat AIDS. In the face of such dark projections for the fate of future generations, macrobiotics represented a small beacon of hope.

From Brazzaville, Michio, Aveline, and the rest of their party went to Germany, Holland, and Yugoslavia to continue to spread their message. Michio's lectures in Yugoslavia, which were arranged by Yugoslav Zlatko Pejic and the Yugloslavian Health, Environment, and Agriculture Committee, drew more than one thousand people in Zagreb and an equal number in Belgrade, many of them medical doctors and scientists.

In May Michio and Aveline visited Japan, Thailand, and Burma. At each place the message was the same one George Ohsawa had given decades before. Now the challenges seemed more severe, yet the Kushis remained ever hopeful, maintaining always that sickness was the mother of health, and that from a handful of tiny grains, a new era of peace could be born.

A v e l i n e   K u s h i ' s
I n t r o d u c t i o n   t o
R e c i p e   S e c t i o n

After nearly forty years of practicing macrobiotics, my ideas about food and cooking have become very simple. Today I have a greater appreciation for food. I respect each vegetable, every grain. I watch the way a squash or a carrot grows and marvel at its wonderful shape. I don't know how it came to be that shape, but it is beautiful.

Food sustains our life. You and your food become one. That is the essence of love.

Our food changes the way we feel and think. It makes us strong or weak. Therefore it affects our direction in life; it guides and influences our physical and spiritual destiny.

We have a deep relationship with everything we eat. Today I see a carrot, a squash, and greens as living beings, as relatives. They are like my brothers and sisters. The vegetable kingdom is my family.

The most important rule in cooking is to respect your food. Treat it with care and love. Be grateful to your food for sustaining you. It is helping you on your spiritual journey.

If you appreciate food and respect it in this way, it will help transform you, and you will get well. You will become very sensitive, and you will understand the effects of each food you eat.

Then you will be able to control your diet very well. It will be easier to control your life.

Grains and vegetables are wonderful things to watch. When we cook them, we watch them change. There are many subtle ways to cook food. We can add more water or use less water; more salt or less salt; more heat, less heat; longer cooking, shorter cooking. There are many ways to cook the same food. And each way changes the food and changes the effects it will have on your body. You can become sensitive to these changes and see which ones help you the most.

Of course, we have recipes that you can learn and begin using immediately. But there is much more to cooking than following a recipe. When someone asks me how long to cook a carrot, I say, Watch and listen to the carrot; it will tell you how long to cook it. Come to understand your food, and it will guide you in proper preparation.

If we do not appreciate our food, it cannot help us. We reject it and it rejects us. It becomes stagnant within us. Here is a very simple way to look at life: Whatever we take in, we must discharge.

All sickness is caused by stagnation. We receive so much every day. In the same way, we must give out. This is the Order of the Universe: to receive and distribute.

All energy must flow freely through us. As each blessing comes to us, we must distribute it to others. This protects us from sickness. If we receive a blessing but do not give out as much in return, energy becomes trapped within us and stagnates. Then sickness comes.

As much as you distribute, that much and more will you receive.

This is the way to happiness. Those who give to others receive more in return and are able to give even more. In this way they become very happy and make others happy, too. Therefore, when you receive a blessing, do not hold it for yourself, but share it with others. That is the essence of health.

RECIPES

These recipes from the files of Aveline Kushi and Wendy Esko are intended to serve as an introduction to cooking the macrobiotic way. Many more delicious and healthful recipes can be found in such cookbooks as *Aveline Kushi's Complete Guide to Macrobiotic Cooking*, written by Aveline Kushi with Alex Jack and published by Warner Books.

GRAIN RECIPES

There are two main methods for cooking grains: pressure-cooking and boiling. Either may be used as explained in the following recipes.

Brown Rice

Pressure-cooking is the preferred method of cooking brown rice the majority of the time. Pressure-cooking allows the rice to cook thoroughly. Pressure-cooked rice is more easily digested, retains more nutrients, is a little less soggy, and has a stronger healing energy than rice cooked by other methods. There are several ways to pressure-cook brown rice; two of the most often used are as follows:

1. *Nonsoaking*. Place the brown rice in a pressure cooker and add the appropriate measure of water. Do not cover. Place on a low flame for approximately 10 minutes. This is a presoaking period, which allows the grain to slowly expand, making it more digestible and sweet. Add the appropriate amount of sea salt, cover, and turn the flame to high. Bring to pressure. When the pressure is up, reduce the flame to medium-low and place a flame deflector under the cooker. Pressure-cook for 50 minutes, remove from the cooker, and serve.

2. *Soaking*. Place the brown rice and water in a pressure cooker and soak overnight or for 6 to 8 hours. Add the appropriate amount of sea salt after the grain has soaked. Cover, place on a high flame, and bring up to pressure. When the pressure is up, reduce the flame to medium-low and cook for 50 minutes.

Basic Pressure-Cooked Brown Rice

2 cups organic brown rice, washed
2½ to 3 cups spring water
Pinch of sea salt per cup of grain

Pressure-cook using one of the above methods. Remove the pressure cooker from the flame and allow the pressure to come down naturally. Remove the cover and allow the rice to sit for 4 to 5 minutes. Remove the rice and place in a wooden serving bowl.

Variations:

- 1½ cups rice and ½ cup barley (soaked overnight)
- 1½ cups rice and ½ cup millet
- 1½ cups rice and ½ cup sweet rice
- 1½ cups rice and ½ cup wheat berries (soaked overnight)
- 1½ cups rice and ½ cup rye (soaked overnight)
- 1½ cups rice and ½ cup hato mugi (pearl barley)
- 1½ cups rice and ½ cup chick-peas (soaked overnight)
- 1½ cups rice and ½ cup aduki beans (soaked overnight)

Sushi

Macrobiotic sushi (made from brown rice and ingredients not chemically treated, and without raw fish) can be eaten frequently as a snack, at parties, or as a handy lunch item. Many types of sushi can be made, using a variety of ingredients.

Vegetable Sushi

Nori
Cooked brown rice
Carrots, cut into strips
Scallion leaves
Umeboshi plum or paste

Roast one side of a sheet of nori over a flame until it turns green, and place on a bamboo sushi mat. Wet both hands with water and spread cooked brown rice evenly on the sheet of nori. Leave about ½ to 1 inch of the top of the nori uncovered with rice, and about ⅛ to ¼ inch of the bottom uncovered.

Slice a carrot into lengthwise strips 8 to 10 inches long and about ¼ inch thick. Place carrot strips in water with a pinch of sea salt. Boil for 2 to 3 minutes. The carrots should be slightly crisp. Remove and allow to cool. Separate the green leaf portion of several scallions from the roots, so that each strip is about 8 to 10 inches in length. Place carrot and scallion strips approximately ½ to 1 inch from the bottom of the sheet of nori. Then lightly spread ¹⁄₁₆ to ⅛ teaspoon puréed umeboshi along the entire length of the carrot and scallion strips.

Roll up the rice and nori, using a sushi mat, pressing the mat firmly against the rice and nori until it is completely rolled up into a round log shape. The vegetables should be centered in the roll. If they are not centered, they were most likely placed too far from the bottom edge of the nori and rice.

Use a very sharp knife and slice the roll into rounds that are about ½ to 1 inch thick. The knife may need to be moistened after each slice. If this is not done, it may not slice properly and may cause the nori to tear.

Arrange rounds on a platter with the cut side up, showing the rice and vegetables, or pack in a lunch box.

Variations: Substitute strips of pickle, deep-fried tofu, cooked tempeh, or root or green vegetables inside the sushi.

Brown Rice and Beans

Brown rice and beans can be prepared in several ways:

1. *Boil* the beans with water to cover for 20 minutes. Add to the rice along with the remaining cooking water and sea salt. Cook as for plain brown rice. This method can be used often with aduki beans.
2. *Soak* the beans 6 to 8 hours or overnight. Discard the soaking water and add the beans to the rice along with water and sea salt. Then pressure-cook as you would plain brown rice.

3. *Dry-roast* the beans. This method is used only with white or black soybeans. Wash the beans, and dry-roast several minutes on a medium flame, stirring constantly. Add the beans to the rice, along with water and sea salt. Pressure-cook as for plain brown rice.

When combining beans with rice, the percentage of beans is usually kept between 10 and 20 percent, with the exception of aduki beans, which can make up as much as 30 percent of the dish. The soaking water from aduki beans can be included as part of the water measurement in cooking. The soaking water from other beans is usually discarded when cooking them with rice.

Sweet Brown Rice and Mochi

Sweet rice is a more glutenous variety of brown rice that is rich in protein and more fatty than regular rice. It is used less often than regular brown rice and may be included several times per week. It can be served plain, cooked with the ingredients listed below, or pounded and made into mochi.

Sweet rice is delicious when cooked in the same way as regular brown rice.

Variations:
- 1 cup sweet rice and 1 cup aduki beans (boiled 15 minutes)
- 1½ cups sweet rice and ½ cup dried chestnuts (dry-roasted until golden and soaked for 10 minutes)
- 1½ cups sweet rice and 1/2 cup dry-roasted black soybeans
- 2 cups sweet rice and 2-inch strip kombu (instead of sea salt)

Mochi (Pounded Sweet Rice)

Mochi is cooked sweet rice that has been pounded for about 30 to 40 minutes or more, with a wooden pestle, until it becomes sticky. It is then dried for 2 to 3 days.

Mochi can be purchased prepackaged in most natural foods stores. To serve, cut into small squares and dry-roast in a skillet until slightly browned on both sides, at which point the mochi puffs up slightly.

Mochi may also be steamed, baked, broiled, pan-fried in oil, deep-fried, or added to soups and stews. Mochi may be eaten with a variety of toppings, including tamari soy sauce, warm brown rice syrup, or toasted soybean flour (kinako). Mochi can also be dry-roasted or toasted and placed in miso soup.

Pressure-Cooked Millet and Vegetables

2 cups millet, washed
2½ to 3 cups water
1 cup hard winter squash, cut in 1-inch chunks
½ cup carrots, sliced in chunks
¼ cup cabbage, sliced in 1-inch squares
Pinch of sea salt per cup of millet

Place all ingredients in a pressure cooker, cover, and bring to pressure. Reduce the flame to medium-low and cook for about 15 to 20 minutes. Remove and allow the pressure to come down. Remove the cover and place the millet in a wooden serving bowl. Garnish and serve.

Udon with Vegetables and Kuzu Sauce

1 package udon (8 oz.), cooked
3 shiitake mushrooms, soaked, destemmed, and sliced
½ cup onions, sliced in ¼-inch-thick wedges
½ cup carrots, sliced on a thin diagonal
¼ cup celery, sliced on a thin diagonal
1 cup broccoli, sliced in small flowerettes
1 cup tofu, cubed and pan-fried until golden
1 strip kombu, 3 to 4 inches long, soaked
2½ cups water
3 tablespoons kuzu,* diluted in 3 tablespoons of water
1½ to 2 tablespoons tamari soy sauce
Grated ginger (optional) for garnish
Sliced scallions for garnish

Place the water, shiitake, and kombu in a pot and bring to a boil. Cover and simmer 4 to 5 minutes. Remove the kombu and set aside for future use. Continue to cook the shiitake for another 5 to 7 minutes. Add the onions, carrots, celery, tofu, and broccoli. Cover, reduce the flame to medium, and simmer until the vegetables are tender but still slightly crisp and brightly colored. Reduce the flame to low and add the diluted kuzu, stirring constantly to prevent lumping. When thick, add the tamari soy sauce for a mild salt taste and simmer 2 to 3 minutes. Place the cooked noodles in individual serving bowls and pour the vegetable-kuzu sauce over them. Garnish with a dab of fresh grated ginger and a few sliced scallions, and serve hot.

*Kuzu is derived from the kudzu or kuzu plant, which grows prevalently throughout much of the United States. It is used as a thickening agent for sauces, stews, and gelatins.

SOUP RECIPES

Basic Vegetable Miso Soup

3 to 4 teaspoons puréed barley miso (mugi)
Sliced scallions for garnish
4 to 5 cups water
½ cup wakame, washed, soaked, and sliced
2 cups onions, sliced in thin half-moons

Place the water in a pot and bring to a boil. Add the wakame, reduce the flame to medium-low, cover, and simmer for 3 to 4 minutes. Add the onions, cover, and simmer another 2 to 4 minutes until the onions and wakame are tender. Reduce the flame to very low and add the puréed miso. Simmer another 2 to 3 minutes. Place in individual serving bowls and garnish with a few sliced scallions. Serve hot.

Kombu may be substituted for wakame. Simply soak for 3 to 4 minutes, slice in very thin matchsticks, and simmer for 5 to 10 minutes before adding the vegetables; or leave whole, simmer for 3 to 5 minutes, and remove.

Variations:
- Carrot, onion, cabbage, and wakame or kombu
- Daikon and wakame or kombu
- Daikon, shiitake, and wakame or kombu
- Daikon, celery, wakame or kombu, and parsley garnish
- Squash, onion, and wakame or kombu
- Celery, onion, scallion, and toasted nori garnish
- Carrot, onion, wakame or kombu, and tofu cubes
- Onion, shiitake, kombu, and parsley garnish
- Turnip, carrot, wakame or kombu
- Wakame, onion, and toasted mochi
- Sweet corn, onion, and wakame or kombu

Lentil Soup

1 cup whole-wheat elbow pasta, cooked, rinsed, and drained
¼ cup chopped parsley
1 cup green lentils, washed
1 strip kombu, 4 or 5 inches long, washed, soaked, and diced
½ cup onions, diced
½ cup carrots, diced
¼ cup celery, diced
2 tablespoons burdock, diced
4 to 5 cups water
¼ to ½ teaspoon sea salt
tamari soy sauce to taste (optional)

Place the kombu, onions, celery, carrots, and burdock in the pot. Set the lentils on top. Cook as above. When 80 percent done, add the sea salt and cook another 20 minutes. Add the cooked pasta and the chopped parsley. Cook another 5 minutes or so. You may add a little tamari soy sauce for a mild salt taste, if desired, at the same time you add the pasta.

Variations: Vegetables other than those in this recipe may also be used. You may also add ¼ cup soaked barley to this soup, letting it cook with the lentils from the beginning.

Koi-ko-ku (Carp-Burdock-Miso Soup)

1 small fresh carp
Burdock (same in weight as carp), shaved
½ to 1 cup *used* bancha twigs,* wrapped and tied tightly in a
    cheesecloth sack
½ to 1 tablespoon fresh grated ginger
Dark sesame oil (optional)
Puréed barley miso to taste
Water
Sliced scallions for garnish

Ask the fish seller to carefully remove the gallbladder and the
yellow bitter bone (thyroid) and leave the rest of the fish intact.
This includes the head, fins, tail, and scales. Next, ask him to
cut the fish into chunks. He may even remove the eyes, if you
wish. Wash the carp and set aside.

   Place a small amount of dark sesame oil in a pressure cooker
and heat up. Add the shaved burdock, and sauté for 2 to 3
minutes. Place the cheesecloth sack filled with used bancha
twigs on top of the burdock. The tea twigs will help to soften
the hard bones of the carp. Do not use fresh unused twigs, as
they will make the soup taste very bitter. Set the carp on top of
the burdock and twigs. Add enough water to cover the carp and
burdock. Place the cover on the pressure cooker and bring up
to pressure. Reduce the flame to medium-low and cook for 1½
to 2 hours. Remove from the flame and allow the pressure to
come down. Remove the cover, add enough puréed miso for a
mild salt taste (½ to 1 teaspoon puréed barley miso per cup of

*Bancha tea is derived from tea bushes that grow widely in Japan. It is a calming,
soothing tea, with only the slightest trace of caffeine. It can be drunk any time during
the day or night. See the Bancha Twig Tea recipe on page 250.

soup), and add the ginger. Reduce the flame to low and simmer until the bones are soft. Place in serving bowls and garnish with sliced scallions.

Carp soup is very strong and is best eaten in small volume. One cup at a time, daily, for two or three days is sufficient in most cases. If taken in larger quantities, it may cause cravings for fruits, liquids, sweets, or other strong yin foods.

Carp soup can be stored in a tightly sealed glass jar in the refrigerator for about 5 to 7 days. However, if frozen, it loses freshness and energy.

Variation: For those with restricted oil intakes, water-sauté the burdock instead of using oil. Carp soup may be boiled instead of pressure-cooked, for 4 to 6 hours, until the bones are soft. As liquid evaporates during boiling, add a little more water.

If carp is not available, you may substitute freshwater trout. Have the insides removed and leave the rest of the trout intact. If burdock is not available, you may substitute carrots, sliced in matchsticks. (Half burdock and half carrots can also be used.) If you use trout, the time needed for pressure-cooking is 50 to 60 minutes. After seasoning with puréed miso and grated ginger, simmer for several more minutes on a low flame. Garnish and serve hot.

Note: In this particular dish a small amount of oil is used for the purpose of softening all bones and high mineral textures of the fish. For persons with serious illness, oil is permissible with this dish.

VEGETABLE RECIPES

Steamed Greens

This particular dish may be eaten daily or often. To prepare, take greens such as turnip, daikon, carrot tops, kale, parsley, watercress, collards, cabbage, Chinese cabbage, radish tops, and the like. Wash and slice them, and place in a steamer or in a small amount of boiling water. Cover and steam several minutes until tender but still bright green.

If you are steaming several types of vegetables, it is best to do each separately to ensure even, proper cooking. They may be mixed after cooking. Also, the stems of green vegetables are often harder than the leafy portion and are best steamed separately, or at least chopped finely before steaming.

It is convenient that a steamer is used for this cooking. Steaming time is about 2 to 3 minutes, depending on the amount and thickness of vegetables.

You may save the water from steaming for use as a soup stock or as a base for a vegetable sauce that can be thickened with kuzu and lightly seasoned with sea salt, tamari soy sauce, or puréed miso. Serve over the vegetables.

Boiled (Blanched) Kale (or Other Greens)

In Japan, this style of cooking is called *ohitashi*. Wash the kale and either leave whole or slice. Place 2 to 3 inches of water in a pot and bring to a boil. Place the kale in the water, cover, and boil 1 to 2 minutes, until deep green but slightly crisp. Remove, drain, and place in a serving bowl.

Boiled (Blanched) Salad

This dish can also be served daily or often. Many kinds of boiled salad can be prepared simply by varying the combination of vegetables or the type of dressing served with the salad. Boiled salad can be served with or without dressing. The following is an example of boiled salad:

2 tablespoons celery, sliced on a thin diagonal
Water
1 cup Chinese cabbage, washed and sliced on a diagonal
1 cup watercress, washed and left whole
¼ cup carrots, sliced in matchsticks

Place 2 to 3 inches of water in a pot and bring to a boil. Place the Chinese cabbage in the pot, cover, and boil for 1 to 2 minutes, or until tender but still a little crisp. Remove, place in a strainer, and allow to drain and cool. Next, place the carrots in the boiling water, cover, and simmer for 1 minute or so. Remove, drain, and allow to cool. Next do the celery, and then the watercress. After draining the watercress, you may slice it in 1-inch lengths. Place all the cooked vegetables in a serving bowl and mix. Serve plain or with a dressing.

Variations:
• Kale, carrot, cabbage, and onion
• Celery and carrot
• Watercress, Chinese cabbage, and sliced red radish
• Daikon, carrot, Chinese cabbage, and turnip greens
• Broccoli, carrot, onion, and cabbage

Note: When making boiled salad, it is best to cook each vegetable separately in the same water. Cook the vegetables with the mildest tastes first, such as onions, daikon, or Chinese cabbage. Then do the stronger-tasting ones like celery, burdock, and watercress.

Salad Dressing Suggestions

1. Purée 1 umeboshi plum, or 1 teaspoon umeboshi paste,* with ½ cup of water in a suribachi.†(Chopped parsley, scallions, or roasted sesame seeds may also be blended in for variety.)

2. Dilute ½ teaspoon barley miso in ½ cup warm water and add about ½ to 1 teaspoon brown rice vinegar. Mix.

3. Dilute 1 teaspoon tamari with ½ cup water and a small amount of chopped parsley. Mix.

4. Lightly sprinkle a desired macrobiotic condiment on the salad.

Nishime

Nishime is another method of boiling and is sometimes referred to as "waterless cooking" because of the low volume of water used. Root or round-shaped vegetables are mostly used, cut in large chunks or rounds. The vegetables are placed in a very small amount of water and cooked on a low flame for 35 to 40 minutes or so. A heavy stainless-steel pot with a heavy cover is recommended for this style of cooking. Pan-fried, deep-fried, or fresh tofu and tempeh may be cooked with the vegetables, as well as dried tofu, seitan,‡ or fu.**

---

*Umeboshi plums are pickled plums grown and pickled in Japan. They provide a strong alkalizing effect on the stomach and are recommended as a substitute for pharmaceutical alkalizers. Umeboshi plums can be used to enhance the taste of rice and other grains and are especially good as a preservative and condiment in rice balls.

†A suribachi is a mortar bowl with a serrated edge used to grind food with a pestle. It is particularly convenient when grinding sesame seeds, kombu seaweed, and other foods to make condiments for grain.

‡Seitan is made from the gluten of wheat. It is usually combined with shoyu or tamari soy sauce to create a hearty, meaty food that is very high in protein.

**Fu is made from the gluten of wheat. Fu is lighter and less "meaty" than seitan. Fu isn't made with the soy sauce or tamari as seitan is, and therefore has only small amounts of sodium.

Nishime cooking produces a very sweet flavor and soft texture and, because of the slow, peaceful cooking process, imparts relaxing and calming energy. It may be used 2 to 4 times per week on average.

¼ cup turnips, sliced in thick chunks
1 strip kombu, washed, soaked, and cut into 1-inch squares
1 cup daikon, sliced in 1-inch-thick rounds
½ cup carrots, sliced in chunks
1 cup buttercup or butternut squash, or Hokkaido pumpkin,
    sliced in large chunks
¼ cup burdock, sliced on a thick diagonal
¼ cup fresh lotus root, sliced in ¼-inch-thick rounds
1 cup cabbage, sliced in 2-inch-thick chunks
Water
Pinch of sea salt
Tamari soy sauce

Place the kombu on the bottom of the pot and add about ½ inch of water. Layer the vegetables on top of the kombu in the following order: daikon, turnips, squash, carrots, lotus root, burdock, and cabbage. Add a pinch of sea salt, cover, and bring to a boil. Reduce the flame to low and simmer for 30 to 35 minutes or until the vegetables are soft and sweet. Add several drops of tamari soy sauce, cover, and simmer for another 5 minutes or so until almost all remaining liquid is gone. Mix the vegetables to coat them evenly with the sweet cooking liquid that remains. Place in a serving bowl.

Variations:
• Carrot, cabbage, burdock, and kombu
• Carrot, lotus root, burdock, and kombu
• Daikon, shiitake, and kombu
• Turnip, shiitake, and kombu
• Onion, cabbage, winter squash, and kombu
• Onion, shiitake, and kombu
• Daikon and kombu

Note: Root vegetables retain their shape even when cooked for a long period. However, squash may dissolve if it is cooked too long and should therefore be added after the other vegetables have cooked for a time.

Dried Daikon and Kombu

This dish can be eaten approximately 2 to 3 times per week; 1 cup per meal is usually sufficient. This is a kind of nitsuke style of cooking.

½ cup dried daikon, rinsed, soaked 10 minutes, and sliced
1 strip kombu, 4 inches long, soaked, and sliced in thin
     matchsticks
Tamari soy sauce
Water

Place the kombu in a heavy skillet or pot, and add the dried daikon. Include enough kombu soaking water to half or three-quarters cover the daikon. Cover, bring to a boil, and reduce the flame to medium-low. Simmer for 30 to 40 minutes until soft and sweet. Add a small amount of tamari soy sauce for a mild taste, cover, and continue to cook several minutes until all liquid is gone.

Variations:
• Dried daikon, kombu, shiitake
• Dried daikon, kombu, carrots, onion

Kinpira Sautéing

This style of cooking combines elements of sautéing and boiling and is similar to braising. It is used mostly for root vegetables. Vegetables are thinly sliced, cut in matchsticks (or, in the case of burdock, shaved), and then sautéed for several minutes in a small amount of sesame oil. (Those with restricted oil intakes may water-sauté instead.) A small amount of water is then added to half cover the vegetables or lightly cover the bottom of the skillet. The vegetables are then covered and cooked on a medium-low flame until about 80 percent done. A small amount of tamari soy sauce can be added for a mild salt taste, and the vegetables are covered again and cooked for another several minutes. The cover is then removed, and the remaining liquid is cooked away. (This style of cooking is also used for arame or hijiki sea vegetables.)

Carrot and Burdock Kinpira

1 cup burdock, shaved
1 cup carrots, sliced in matchsticks
Water
Tamari soy sauce
Dark sesame oil (optional)

Place a small amount of dark sesame oil in a skillet and heat up. Add the burdock, and sauté for 2 to 3 minutes. Set the carrots on top of the burdock. Do not mix. Add enough water to lightly cover the bottom of the skillet, and bring to a boil. Cover and reduce the flame to medium-low. Cook until the vegetables are about 80 percent done, perhaps 7 to 10 minutes. Add a few drops of tamari soy sauce, cover, and cook for several more minutes. Remove the cover and cook until all remaining liquid evaporates.

Variations:
- Carrot, burdock, and dried tofu
- Carrot, burdock, and lotus root
- Carrot, onion, and lotus root
- Onion, turnip, and lotus root
- Carrot, onion, burdock, and seitan

Note: These dishes may be eaten 2 to 3 times per week, averaging about ½ cup per serving.

Aduki Beans with Kombu and Squash

1 cup aduki beans, soaked 4 to 6 hours
1 cup hard winter squash, cubed (use acorn, buttercup, or
    butternut squash, or Hokkaido pumpkin; carrots or
    parsnips may be substituted if squash is not available)
1 strip kombu, 1 to 2 inches long, soaked and diced
Water
Sea salt

Place the kombu on the bottom of a pot. Set the squash on top. Place the aduki beans on top of the squash. Add water to just cover the squash. Bring to a boil, cover, and reduce the flame to low. Simmer until about 80 percent done. Season with ¼ teaspoon of sea salt per cup of beans, cover, and continue to cook another 15 to 20 minutes until soft and creamy.

Variations:
- 1 cup aduki beans, ½ cup lotus seeds, and kombu
- 1 cup aduki beans, ½ cup dried chestnuts, and kombu
- 1 cup aduki beans, ¼ cup soaked wheat berries, and kombu
- 1 cup aduki beans, ¼ cup dried apples, 1 tablespoon
    raisins, and kombu (can be used as a sweet dessert)

Chick-peas and Vegetables

1 cup chick-peas, soaked 6 to 8 hours or overnight
1 cup carrots, sliced in chunks
½ cup celery, sliced on a thick diagonal
1 strip kombu, 1 to 2 inches long, soaked and diced
Water
Sea salt or puréed barley miso

Place the kombu, celery, carrots, and chick-peas in a pot and add water to just cover. Prepare using either the nishime or kinpira methods described previously. When 80 percent done, season with tamari soy sauce, sea salt, or puréed barley miso. If boiling, chick-peas may take 3 to 4 hours.

Variations:
• Carrot, onion, and toasted nori squares
• Season with a small amount of umeboshi vinegar instead of tamari soy sauce
• Season with a pinch of sea salt instead of tamari soy sauce or umeboshi vinegar
• Water-sauté the vegetables instead of using oil

Tempeh with Sauerkraut and Cabbage

1 cup tempeh, cubed
1 cup green cabbage, shredded
¼ cup sauerkraut, chopped
Small amount of sauerkraut juice
Tamari soy sauce

Heat a skillet and add the tempeh cubes. Place a drop of tamari on each cube and brown slightly. Add the sauerkraut and cabbage. Add enough sauerkraut juice or plain water to half cover the tempeh. Bring to a boil, cover, and reduce the flame to low. Simmer about 20 to 25 minutes. Remove the cover and cook off any remaining liquid.

Variations:
• Tempeh and leek
• Tempeh, scallion, and ginger juice
• Tempeh and onion, with parsley garnish
• Season with tamari soy sauce or a little umeboshi paste or plum instead of sauerkraut juice

SEA VEGETABLE RECIPES

Arame with Carrots and Onions

1 ounce dried arame, rinsed, drained, and allowed to sit 3 to 5 minutes
½ cup onions, sliced in thin half-moons
½ cup carrots, sliced in matchsticks
Dark sesame oil
Water
Tamari soy sauce

Lightly brush dark sesame oil in a skillet and heat up. Place the onions in the skillet and sauté 1 to 2 minutes. Place the sliced carrots on top of the onions. Slice the arame and set on top of the carrots. Do not mix. Add enough water to just cover the vegetables but not the arame, and a very small amount of tamari. Bring to a boil, reduce the flame to medium-low, and cover. Simmer for about 35 to 40 minutes. Lightly season with a few drops of tamari for a mild salt taste. Cover and cook another 5 to 7 minutes. Remove the cover and continue to cook until almost all liquid is gone. Mix and cook off remaining liquid. Garnish and serve.

Variations:
• Arame, onion, and lotus root
• Arame, onion, carrot, and tempeh (plain or fried)
• Arame with roasted sesame seed garnish
• Arame and dried daikon
• Arame, onion, and sweet corn
• Water-sauté the vegetables

Quick Tamari Soy Sauce Vegetable Pickles

Thin slice a variety of root or ground vegetables and place in a glass jar. Cover with a mixture of ½ water and ½ tamari soy sauce. Shake and cover the jar with clean cotton cheesecloth. Allow to sit in a cool place for 2 to 3 hours. Remove and serve, or if too salty, rinse quickly and serve.

COOKED-FRUIT RECIPES

Stewed Fruit with Kuzu

2 cups apple juice or water (or half and half)
1 cup sliced apples or pears
1 tablespoon raisins
Pinch of sea salt
3 heaping teaspoons kuzu

Place the raisins, apple juice or water, and pinch of sea salt in a pot and bring to a boil. Reduce the flame to medium-low, cover, and simmer until the apples are soft. Turn the flame down low. Dilute the kuzu in a small amount of water and pour it into the apple mixture, stirring constantly to prevent lumping. When thick, simmer 1 minute. Remove and serve.

Variations:
• Use other northern varieties of fruit
• Use ½ cup dried fruit, soaked and sliced

Amasake Pudding

1 pint amasake*
1 cup apples or pears
3 teaspoons kuzu, diluted

Place the apples and amasake in a saucepan and bring to a boil. Reduce the flame to medium-low and simmer until the fruit is soft. Reduce the flame to low, add the diluted kuzu, stirring constantly to prevent lumping. Simmer 1 minute or so until thick. Remove and serve.

*Amasake is a sweet drink made from sweet brown rice, water, and rice koji, a friendly bacteria used to ferment the sweet rice to give it a creamy consistency and make it rich in digestive enzymes.

Variations:
- Use other northern varieties of fruit
- Use ½ cup dried fruit, soaked, and sliced
- Omit fruit entirely and prepare plain
- Add 1 teaspoon of prepared, instant grain coffee to the amasake

Kanten

Agar-agar flakes (follow package instructions for amount of liquid)
Pinch of sea salt
4 cups water
2 cups dried apples, soaked and sliced

Place the water, sea salt, dried apples, and kanten (agar-agar) flakes in a pot. Bring to a boil, reduce the flame to low, cover, and simmer until the apples are soft. Remove and pour the apples and liquid into a dish. Refrigerate or place in a cool place until jelled. Kanten is usually ready to serve in 45 to 60 minutes. Slice or spoon into serving dishes.

BEVERAGE RECIPES

Bancha Twig Tea (Kukicha)

Place 1 tablespoon of bancha twigs in 1 quart of water and bring to a boil. Reduce the flame to low. Simmer 1 to 3 minutes for a mild taste or up to 15 minutes for a stronger tea. Drink while hot.

Sweet Vegetable Broth

½ cup green cabbage, sliced very thin
2 quarts water
½ cup carrots, diced
½ cup onions, diced
½ cup winter squash, sliced very thin

Place all ingredients in a pot, cover, and bring to a boil. Reduce the flame to low and simmer for 10 to 15 minutes. Remove from flame and strain off the sweet broth. Drink 1 cup or so. Store in a glass jar in the refrigerator and heat up as needed. Save the cooked vegetables from making the broth and use in soups.

APPENDIXES

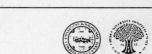

Boston University School of Medicine
at Boston University Medical Center

80 East Concord Street
Boston, Massachusetts 02118
(617) 638- 4274/4298
Department of Microbiology

Michio Kushi
62 Buckminster Rd.
Brookline, Mass. 02146   January 15, 1986

Dear Michio,

The results of our ongoing study of men with AIDS who are macrobiotic
are encouraging. We have been studing the men sequentially since May 1984
to follow certain immune parameters. At present the data suggest a stabilization of the % T_4 positive cells and lymphocyte number in about 50% of the
group. The general pattern in people with KS is a steady decline in both
%T_4 and total lymphocyte number. This is thought to be a significant indicator
of morbidity. Therefore the ability to stabilize these parameters, in so
large a proportion of our study group, is a hopeful sign.

Elinor M. Levy, Ph.D
Associate Professor
Department of Microbiology

John C. Beldekas Ph.D.
Research Associate
Department of Microbiology

PATIENTS WITH KAPOSI'S SARCOMA WHO OPT FOR ALTERNATIVE THERAPY

Elinor M. Levy, J. C. Beldekas,
P. H. Black, and L. H. Kushi

Dept. of Microbiology,
Boston University School of Medicine, Boston, MA, USA
and Division of Epidemiology,
University of Minnesota, Minneapolis, MN, USA

INTRODUCTION

We have been studying changes in immune parameters in a group of men with Kaposi's sarcoma who are following a vegetarian (macrobiotic) diet designed by Michio Kushi and his associates.

We have been sequentially studying, *since May 1984*, immune function in a group of men with Kaposi's sarcoma who had chosen to forego conventional medical treatment. They are following a vegetarian (macrobiotic) diet. A preliminary report of the first 10 men to enter the study appeared in Lancet II; 223, 1985. The study has been expanded to include 24 men. For those subjects with more than one set of determinations, the data indicate the percentage and number of lymphocyte subsets are reasonably stable or are increasing over time.

The percentage of T4 cells on first measurement was 24.2 ± 3.1 (mean ± SE) versus 20.3 ± 4.3 for the most recent measurement, an average of 11.7 ± 1.9 months later (n = 10). At the same time the percentage of T8 cells went from 28.7 ± 2.9 to 32.3 ± 3.8. The ability of patient cells to form T cell colonies in agar increased from 46.9 ± 9.6 to 63.8 ± 14.3 over a period of 9.3 ± 1.6 months (n = 14). Lymphocyte number also increased from 1661 ± 182 to 1933 ± 174 over a 12.4 ± 3.1 month interval (n = 10). Mitogenesis in response to PHA expressed relative to a healthy control decreased from 83.3 ± 14.5 to 54.2 ± 12.5 over a 7.9 ± 1.0 month interval (n = 14). The average survival for those who have died has been 25.0 ± 4.2 months (n = 6). The relative stability of lymphocyte number and distribution in this group as compared to reports of other groups suggests the possibility that certain treatments may contribute to the decrease in lymphocyte number associated with the progression of AIDS.

SURVIVAL

For the initial cohort of men, the average survival time for those who have died (6/10) is 25 months. The average time from diagnosis for those now living (4/10) is 37 months.

LYMPHOCYTE NUMBER VS. TIME
IN PEOPLE WITH KS [p<.003]

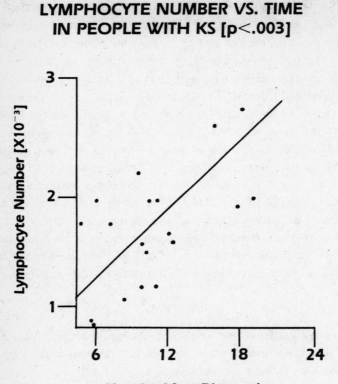

The average calculated lymphocyte number/mm^3 increases from 1122 at diagnosis to 2584 2 years later. The calculation is based on all the data points available.

Changes in Lymphocyte Number for Individuals with KS on a Macrobiotic Diet

INITIAL	WITHIN 2 YEARS OF DIAGNOSIS		SINCE DIAGNOSIS	
LYMPH #	LYMPH #	Δ T	LYMPH #	Δ T
1368	1800	19.2	2280	29.1
1575	1935	23.0	2500	31.1
1400	2698	13.9	2698	13.9
1530	1575	4.6	1575	4.6
1677	1920	5.7	1920	5.7
2760	2375	9.4	2375	9.4
836	1150	6.4	1150	6.4
1344	1918	11.2	1918	11.2
2560	—		1850	9.9
1564	—		1064	3.0
1161 ± 182	1921 ± 166	11.7 ± 6.6	1933 ± 173	12.4 ± 3.1

Lymphocyte number increases for 7/8 men for whom more than one measurement within two years of diagnosis is available. Lymphocyte number increases for 7/10 men over the entire period of observation. Time is expressed in months between.

Changes in Immune Parameters in Men with Kaposi's Sarcoma on a Macrobiotic Diet

| | WITHIN 2 YEARS OF DIAGNOSIS | | | | SINCE DIAGNOSIS | | | |
	INITIAL	MOST RECENT	N	TIME MONTHS	INITIAL	MOST RECENT	N	TIME MONTHS
%T4	20.2 ± 1.7*	20.9 ± 4.7	7	7.1 ± 1.7	24.2 ± 3.1	20.3 ± 4.3	10	11.7 ± 1.9
%T8	31.8 ± 2.8	37.3 ± 4.0	7	7.1 ± 1.7	28.7 ± 2.9	32.3 ± 3.5	10	11.7 ± 1.9
Mitogen (% control)	77.4 ± 13.9	49.7 ± 8.3	12	6.5 ± 1.0	83.3 ± 14.5	54.2 ± 12.5	14	9.2 ± 1.7
T-CFC (% control)	40.5 ± 8.9	37.6 ± 7.6	12	6.5 ± 1.0	46.9 ± 9.6	63.8 ± 14.3	14	9.3 ± 2.6
Lymphocyte number	1561 ± 193	1921 ± 165	8	10.4 ± 2.2	1661 ± 182	1933 ± 174	10	12.4 ± 3.1

*Mean ± SE

Correlations with Time after Diagnosis and T-CFC for Men with KS Who Are Macrobiotic

	WITHIN 2 YEARS OF DIAGNOSIS			SINCE DIAGNOSIS		
	R	P	N	R	P	N
Lymph# vs time	0.6595	0.0005	24	0.3007	0.084	34
T4% vs time	0.1562	0.385	33	0.5170	0.0002	46
T8% vs time	−0.3424	0.048	34	0.2240	0.130	47
T4/T8 vs time	0.2592	0.139	34	0.4318	0.002	48
T4# vs time	0.3928	0.064	23	0.4546	0.008	33
T8# vs time	0.1915	0.370	24	−0.0015	0.994	34
Lymph# vs T-CFC	0.5724	0.008	20	0.3567	0.058	29
T4% vs T-CFC	0.4840	0.017	24	0.5853	0.0002	36
T4# vs T-CFC	0.4937	0.032	19	0.6155	0.0005	28

R = Pearson correlation coefficient
N = All data points

CONCLUSION

1. Lymphocyte number increases over the first two years from diagnosis with Kaposi's sarcoma in men who are following a macrobiotic diet. A linear regression analysis model predicts that lymphocyte number becomes normal within this two year period.

2. During this time period the percentage of T4 cells does not change. The percentage of T8 cells possibly decreases.

3. These results compare favorably with those from any of the medical treatments reported.

4. There are several possible explanations for these positive findings including:

    A) The macrobiotic diet and/or life-style is of benefit to men with Kaposi's sarcoma.

    B) The decision to become and remain macrobiotic selects for men with a better prognosis.

III International Conference on Acquired Immunodeficiency Syndrome (AIDS)

June 1-5, 1987—Washington, DC USA

Official Abstract Submission Form

ONLY THIS OFFICIAL FORM IS ACCEPTABLE (no photocopies) as the original submission. However, 5 copies on white bond paper should be submitted with this original abstract form.

1. Type within blue lines: Title, Authors' Names (6 or less), Affiliations, City, State, Country and Abstract. (Underline name to indicate presenter; if there are more than 6 authors, type et al. to indicate additional authors. Do not include more than 6 authors' names. Limit abstracts to 250 words—includes author information.)

Patients with Kaposi's sarcoma who opt for alternative therapy: immune and psychological measures.
ELINOR M.LEVY*, M.COTTRELL**,L.H.KUSHI***,and P.H.BLACK*,*Boston University School of Medicine,Boston,MA,**Fashion Institute of Technology,NY,***University of Minnesota,Minneapolis,MN.

Twenty ~~four~~ men who have chosen a holistic approach to their diagnosis of Kaposi's sarcoma have been studied sequentially. They are all following a macrobiotic regimen. The median survival for the 8 men who have died is 19 months (range 5-46 months). None of the surviving members of the cohort have required hospitalization. One has required local radiation. Four are alive 3 or more years after diagnosis. Contrary to what might be expected, the number of lymphocytes in the group has increased with time over the first 3 years after diagnosis ($r=0.474,p=0.006$). The number of T4 cells increased over the first 2 years after diagnosis ($r=0.458,p$ 0.03). The percentage of T8 cells was unchanged ($r=-0.06,p=0.69$). A subset of approximately 1/3 of these patients have filled out psychological questionnaires,including the Beck Depression Inventory (BDI) and the McNair's Profile of Moods Survey (POMS). Preliminary data suggests these men are generally less depressed (median BDI score 10, range 1-28),less anxious (median POMS Tension score 4,range 3-6),and feel more energetic (median POMS Vigor score 23,range 8-32) than has been reported for other cohorts of men with AIDS. The psychological profile associated with this group is hypothesized to have a beneficial effect on the clinical course of their disease.

2. Category submitted under (see reverse side)

General Category ___Psychosocial_____ Code __F__

Sub-Category ___Other_____ Code __9__

3. Preference: Oral presentation ___X___ Poster Presentation _____

4. Provide the following about the presenter:

Name of presenter ___Elinor M. Levy___

Affiliation/Institution ___Boston University School of Medicine___

Mailing address (Business) ___80 E. Concord St.___

___Boston, MA 02118___

Telephone No. (include area code) ___617-638-4274___

5. Mail this original Official Abstract Submission Form and 5 copies to:

Scientific Program Committee
III International Conference on AIDS
655 15th Street, N.W., Suite 300
Washington, DC 20005 USA

> ABSTRACTS MUST BE RECEIVED
> NO LATER THAN FEBRUARY 1, 1987

6. Complete and return the Acknowledgement Card with your abstract if you wish to receive confirmation of receipt of your abstract(s).

REVIEWERS USE ONLY: A _____ R _____ Score _____ Oral _____ Poster _____
COMMENTS:

Testimony for the Presidential Commission on the
Human Immunodeficiency Virus Epidemic
February 20, 1988
New York, NY

Elinor M. Levy, Ph.D.
Associate Professor of Microbiology
Boston University School of Medicine
Boston, MA 02118

Each year we learn a little more about the natural history
of HIV infections. We now know that following infection with
HIV some individuals develop AIDS within a year, while others
remain without any symptoms for at least 7 years. Similarly, we
know that some individuals with Kaposi's sarcoma (KS) die within
months of diagnosis, while others live longer than 6 years. At
this point, however, we have little evidence to explain these dif-
ferences, and therefore are unable to advise the estimated 1–2
million Americans infected with HIV how to maximize their
longevity. Should they change their habits, their diets, their attitudes? There is evidence that suggests that each of these might
influence progression of HIV related diseases.

I will concentrate my remarks on nutrition as a possible
cofactor in HIV related disease. In general, malnutrition is associated with a significantly impaired immune response. The
immune response is also sensitive to deficiencies and excesses
of single nutritional elements, and to the quantity and quality
of fat intake. Nutrition can be shown to affect susceptibility to
a variety of infectious agents, and is implicated in the develop-
ment of cancer. I have been involved in a pilot study of men
with AIDS related diseases who have chosen to follow a macrobiotic regimen. This includes a vegetarian diet, a healthy life-
style, and a sense of hope and control. The large majority report
an improvement in AIDS related symptoms. Additionally, those in
the group with KS also showed an increase in their number of
lymphocytes during the first 3 years after diagnosis, and 6/19 of
these men are alive greater than 3 years after diagnosis with KS.

Research into nutrition as a cofactor for progression of HIV related disease is difficult for several reasons, among them prevailing research priorities, the complexity of study in this area, and certain methodological problems. Research priorities have focused on finding a cure and developing a vaccine, both worthwhile but still elusive goals. Only recently has there been a shift to include education to prevent HIV infection, and an interest by ADAMHA in the role of psychosocial factors, including alcohol and drug abuse, in AIDS progression. The group we have been studying is an example of the likely interrelationship between nutritional, psychosocial, and behavioral choices. Studies must take into account these interrelationships in order to interpret data correctly. Additionally there are methodological problems in accurately assessing nutritional status, particularly if absorption may be a problem.

I would recommend that the NIH foster more of an interest in nutritional and other cofactors through the organization of small workshops to bring together the multidisciplinary talents needed to work out design and methodological issues, and by encouraging research through RFAs. I would recommend that nutritional components be added onto ongoing "natural history" studies, and/or that new studies focusing on psychosocial and nutritional cofactors be encouraged, including those with an intervention design. Finally, I would recommend that NIH create multidisciplinary review committees to properly evaluate these grant applications.

At this time I cannot give an estimated cost for implementing these recommendations, but suggest it would be a modest investment compared to what could be saved in health care and social service costs if onset of debilitating symptoms can be delayed or prevented. Although the state of our knowledge about the factors predisposing to the progression of HIV infection is not extensive, it is extremely likely that cofactors play an important role. There is an urgent need for research in these areas, so that accurate information can be used as a basis for more effective treatment strategies and educating persons at risk.